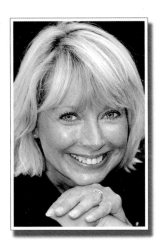

Rhona's *Diary*

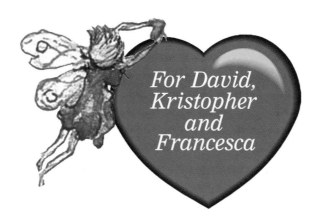

For David,
Kristopher
and
Francesca

Photographs © Archant Regional Ltd, Rhona Damant, OTTTO Holdings (Aust.) Pty Ltd trading as BridgeClimb®, 2005.

The right of Rhona Damant to be identified as author of this work has been asserted in accordance with the Copyright, Designs and Patents Act, 1988.

ISBN 0-9548737-1-8

Printed by Healeys, Unit 10, The Sterling Complex, Farthing Road, Ipswich, Suffolk, IP1 5AP.

Foreword
By Ronan Keating

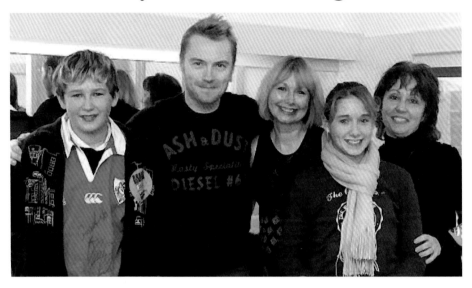

HONOURED: Rhona, her son Kristopher, her daughter Francesca and her friend Laini White meet Ronan Keating before his concert at Wembley Arena in December, 2004

Every time I speak or write about cancer, I cannot help but think of my mother and the pain she went through.

However, through it all she remained our mother, and she was still there smiling when we would turn up at home making sure we had eaten enough and that everything was OK with us. It always amazed us how much strength and pride she had until her last days.

I am truly amazed and feel very humble when I read Rhona's column. To be in her position yet to have come to a stage where she has confronted the disease, almost overcome it, and be pushed right back again is hard enough. But to still have peace with herself and not feel angry, especially that she will not get to see her kids grow up is almost unbelievable. As a parent, that is the hardest thing for anyone to deal with.

I am truly honoured to be able to say a few words about Rhona and she is an inspiration to us all. Someone said that we are remembered by the gifts we leave our children. Well Rhona, you have left the finest gift of all for yours. Love and life.

God Bless you
from

Ronan Keating
November 2004

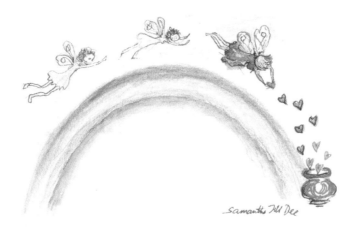

Samantha Jill Dee

Introduction

It was a simple phone call that introduced Rhona Damant into the pages of the *East Anglian Daily Times* and into the lives and hearts of so many of its readers.

Rhona told us that she'd like to tell the story of a mother fighting terminal breast cancer — it was her own story.

Could we find room for it in the paper? Of course we could, and her columns were an instant success.

By turns brave, funny, warm, sharp, always emotional and direct, Rhona's words dragged a taboo blinking into the daylight.

People just didn't talk about the c-word like this, especially publicly, but here was a woman, a mother, laying it all on the line; this is what cancer is, this is how it affects you, your family, your friends, your life.

Her following grew rapidly, and readers started to write in to share their experiences, offer their thoughts and prayers, to suggest treatments and proffer their gifts after reading a unique story told by an extraordinary, vital person who has endured so much but fought back so hard.

The story of this book's title goes a long way to summing up Rhona's approach. It was, to most women, the stuff of nightmares. She was in the office of her consultant and he'd just given her the worst news - that she had breast cancer.

She just burst out laughing, and it took his barked "sit down and stop laughing" command to halt her hilarity and bring matters back to the level of gravitas and solemnity he felt appropriate.

Rhona's Diary is a searingly honest, compelling account of a devastating illness, lit up with shafts of her Northern Irish humour. It may make you laugh, it may make you cry, but you will not finish this book without experiencing something of the emotion that Rhona and her family have been through.

Thank you, Rhona.

**Dominic Castle,
Deputy Editor,
East Anglian Daily Times.**

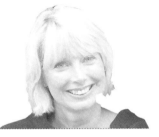

Rhona's
Diary

October 13, 2003: *Busy time will soon take toll*

IT'S amazing what can happen in several days. Firstly Katy (Edwards, EADT feature writer) came to visit to do the article for the paper, followed by photographs being taken of the children, dog and myself in the garden, telephone calls from people I will never know wishing me well, letters of support, friends teasing me about being on the front of the paper, my first session of Reiki, and a close friend taking me to Holkham beach for the day.

We drove for over two hours there and back just to walk on the beach. It might seem a crazy thing to do but it is one of the many things I want to do before I have to say goodbye.

The day was as wonderful as I could have wished for, sunny and bright, but enough chill in the air to make it feel like autumn. We walked for ages along the gorgeous sands, talking and laughing as if it was a normal day, but of course it wasn't. All the time we both knew it was something I would never do again. To know I would never enjoy time here with my family on a beautiful summer day was really very upsetting.

It has been a busy time, but I know it will all very soon take its toll on me and I will need to sleep for ages. I used to feel I should not give into this horrible disease by sleeping. I now know that tiredness is my body's way of telling me it needs some help.

It was during my last visit to the Royal Marsden Hospital in London, when once again the tubes were in (they eventually found a vein that had not collapsed) that I realised cancer is now very much a young person's disease.

As I was enduring my three-hour bone-strengthening drip, which always seems to last all day, I noticed the girl next to me was in her early 20s. My age group appears to be now in the majority rather than the minority. Why is it then that mammograms are still only offered to women over 50 years old? I have raised this question many times with medical professionals, but have never been given a constructive answer.

Recently the age group was extended to women over 70 for this regular scan. Surely women under 50 should be offered this very important screening, especially if there is any family history connection? If I had been offered this when I first discovered my breast lump, then I would not be in the situation I am in today.

As it was, I was told this unusual lump invading my body was part of me. I went home happy, believing it wasn't the dreaded "Big C".

October is Breast Cancer Awareness Month, so, surely, as women are remembering to check for anything different in their bodies, due to the reminders in many magazines and papers, this issue of screening should — once again — be raised with those

'Tiredness is my body's way of telling me it needs help'

1

who make health decisions. We should be asking them to think again about lowering the age. It could help prevent the unnecessary heartbreak of this killer disease and give some children a longer future with their mothers.

There is just one more thing I would like to add - why do perfect women have to model the T-shirts for breast cancer? Hasn't anyone ever thought of the hurt it causes to see this, especially when you are trying to come to terms with a mastectomy, coping with the loss of femininity and not feeling at all as perfect as those who are modelling this important fundraising idea.

I am just about to finish my last cycle of chemotherapy. Fingers crossed, I will have responded, so that when I have my CT scan and MRI in the coming week there will be a little glimmer of hope for myself and my family.

Meantime, life must go on as normal...

Rhona x

....

October 20, 2003: *Battling to keep things normal*

IT has been a mixture of all emotions in the Damant household this week. Having only just bought my children very expensive camera mobile phones so that they can take them when they compete in swimming galas (both swim for Hadleigh Swimming Club) or any other activity which I am now unable to attend due to a failing immune system, my son had his stolen. The person who took it will find it useless to him as I immediately put a block on the phone, but he has now taken away what pleasure I would have had in seeing the photos which Kristopher's friends would have taken of him at various stages of the day.

I try to spend each day under an illusion of "being normal". I am very lucky that I can do this, as I know many cancer sufferers, for all sorts of reasons feel that they have entered a huge dark tunnel without an exit, but I too had my tearful side this week.

It was fortunate for me that both things happened in the same morning, so I was able to feel sad, angry, scared and just about every other feeling that can happen when the realisation hits that cancer is starting to take over my life.

But then I followed the advice of the old saying and picked myself up, brushed myself off and then went out and did what my husband now dreads - had a "lady who lunches" afternoon. (Of course I can't understand myself, being a woman, why David has to always mention the word "bankrupt" when he looks at the calendar every day!)

I expect you are wondering what made me feel like this. It was two little things that broke my heart.

First of all, when I was washing my hair that morning I found that I could not squeeze the shampoo bottle - I had managed during the night to somehow lose most of the power and strength in my right hand.

Although I was told that this would start to happen, I wasn't ready for it just yet. I have since found that now first thing in the morning my hand is really quite useless, but feeling starts to creep back a little during the day.

The second thing was writing David's birthday card. What do you write, on what will probably be the last card that you give to your husband for his birthday?

The tears of that moment, I believe, have been the worst that I have ever shed (but did prove that my mascara was actually waterproof after all!).

When finally my sight became clearer and

also my mind, I knew the only thing to write was "with all my love forever and ever, please always remember that."

Chemo has now finished, but with that my cough is starting to reappear and so is the pain. The scans have taken place along with my bone-drip.

I have just got to be the world's worst needle phobic. I am embarrassed to say that with every needle I have I also need the "wimp" cream, otherwise known as the anaesthetic cream used for babies and children, so it was "freak out" time for me when I was told that my feet would be used soon for canulas as I was quickly running out of veins...oh the joy of chemo!

I will be going to the Marsden soon to see the consultants. I really don't know what I am going to hear, or how I will react to the results. I expect there will be tears whether they are good or bad. To the outside world it will be a normal autumn day with the colours changing and the leaves falling, but to us it will be another day of waiting and hoping that I may be given the chance of just a little while longer to be with my family and many friends.

It is funny really, as I have never watched the beauty of each season, the summer meant so much to me watching the children out every day playing with their friends. The balmy nights which meant I just had to have a really cool beer!

And now the delight of autumn. Strangely enough I never really liked this time of year before, but now I want to enjoy every minute of it.

The thing is, no-one knows what is just around the corner.

Rhona x

....

October 27, 2003: *Against the odds, some good news*

IT was a very long four days of waiting from having my scans to getting the results.

Thankfully, I slept most of the time, which stopped me from worrying. I had even managed to fall asleep during my MRI, which, for those of you who have had experience of this scan, is not an easy thing to do, as it is extremely noisy.

Suddenly, a voice in my headphones was telling me to stop moving or it would ruin the scan - it was then I realised I had been chasing a cat in my sleep!

At last, Monday - results day - arrived. After a restless night I was very tired when our ambulance car picked us up for the journey to London (transport is one of the perks of being terminally ill).

Both David and myself were in a subdued mood. We talked about what we would do on arriving in Brisbane (we are planning a huge family holiday to Australia this Christmas) but really no decisions were made. To be honest, both of us were in limbo.

We had our normal, unappetising Marsden lunch then headed off to outpatients. I became engrossed in a magazine issued in July 1997.

Suddenly, my name was called and I thought all the waiting was over. But a nurse showed David and myself into a side room where we waited for a consultant for 20 minutes. It felt like mental torture.

At last, we were greeted by a doctor who I had only met once before, but who I knew was someone I could talk to and respect.

He shook our hands, smiled at us and said the magic words - "It's good news".

Every emotion ran through me. I didn't know whether to laugh or cry, say thank you or just hold on to his every word, so I did all four. When tumours are present in the brain it is usually difficult to find treatment to break through what is known as the blood brain barrier.

As my initial treatment of having chemo injected into my spine once a week hadn't worked I had been told there was not much hope of a favourable result after my MRI scans.

Guess what? My three tumours have shrunk and it would seem that I have defied all the odds!

This apparently should not happen, so it was quite a miraculous result! The scans also showed less fluid around my lungs, and a slight decrease of cells in my liver. Unfortunately, my spine didn't look too good, so I will now have to have radiotherapy as there is chance of the cancer eating my vertebrae.

My ribs have already been eaten away, which often results in experiencing quite sickening pain.

I am keen to start my treatment soon to stop that from happening on my back. Radiotherapy does not frighten me. I responded very well after my intense course three years ago. I am, however, not looking too forward to all those scary needles leaving "tattoos" engraved on my spine.

I will never know how I have managed to buy myself some more time with David and my "babies" (OK, so they may be 12 and 13 but they will always be just that to me and they will cringe when they read this.) Obviously my trial drug is doing wonders, but I do believe other things have contributed to it as well.

I refuse to think of myself as the cancer patient and try to live as I always have. I believe there is a lot to be said for keeping positive.

Also, I know prayers have been said and candles have been lit for me by so many people, even by some of my daughter's little friends.

My name has apparently even been mentioned in the Vatican, in Rome, by another friend. I have so many people to thank for helping me try to achieve my goal - to still be here next September when my daughter starts senior school.

I have received letters, books and videos from people and help from a lovely gentleman in Bury St Edmunds, who is determined to give me a better quality of life by introducing me to some very special natural products.

Along with the children's memory boxes I have now started a "support box" so that when I have lost the battle my children will always be able to look back and read of all the help and kind thoughts I received from strangers.

For now, we are in the middle of half term and, like any mother, I almost went insane on day one.

Still, I am determined to enjoy it, despite the untidiness of the house, the cries of "I'm bored", the fighting and the staying in pyjamas all day.

Rhona x

November 3, 2003: *One party I m not going to miss*

IT has been a great week with the children, but unfortunately it was over all too quickly.

The highlight of the week was going up to Manchester to visit my best friend, Louise, and her family, with a greeting from their little son George: "Hi Auntie Rhona, superstar." (I send both Louise and another very close friend who I have known since I was eight, Elizabeth, who lives in York along with John, her husband, a copy of the EADT each week.) It does make me smile to think that George now considers me to be "famous" but, deep down, he doesn't really understand why.

Louise is helping me to organise my funeral as, when the time comes, I don't believe that David will be able to cope with my death. I know who I want to carry me into the church (all of whom I have now asked), the music, hymns and, of course, not forgetting my request of single lilies, with any donations to the hospice which I now attend.

We even talked about my wake, but then I decided I would like to be there, so we are planning a "pre-wake party" in the spring so that I can enjoy myself, too. (Is this completely MAD? Of course it is, but my friends mean too much to me to let them be sad over my departure, so I want them all to remember the humorous side of me!)

Once that was over our enjoyment began! We went to Alton Towers for the Hallowe'en spectacular - the four children and three adults had an absolutely brilliant time on the rides. The fourth adult - me - well, I had a great time on the "Swans"!

Our time in the North was just what we all needed, to get away from reality and forget what is really going on in our lives, and we did just that.

I have now been put on a further two cycles of chemo but have been told that, after that, it would make me feel very ill so, in the New Year, I hope I will be put on to a different type of chemo. And, if I have the hormone, HER2 positive, present in my body, then I may be allowed the new drug Herceptin which, according to every detail I have found to read, can give an advanced breast cancer sufferer an extra year of life, so please, please let me have that hormone.

I still have not heard from the radiotherapy department at the Marsden. Although I was told I would have it this side of Christmas it is now looking unlikely that I will finish the treatment before we go Down Under as I still haven't even had the appointment to be marked up (the tiny tattoos which will be inked around my spine).

This is beginning to upset me a little as this treatment would take away some of the pain which I experience very frequently in my spine and neck.

I would like to be as pain-free as possible on our holiday, but time is starting to run out on me, so let's hope that, if I need one, there will be a bright-coloured Australian wheelchair available! I have a wonderful Macmillan nurse who I see regularly. She is always there when I need questions answered or help on various things.

'*Louise is helping me organise my funeral*'

If I can't get answers from the hospital I know that she will, so it is so assuring that anything which I need for our trip she will help me sort it out.

When I was diagnosed in 1999, I refused to have a Macmillan nurse as I can remember when my mum was ill, nurses coming to our home meant only one thing ... death.

It frightened me four years ago when this was offered to me, as bad memories came flooding back, so I'm not sure why it seemed to be all right this time to have a nurse, but whatever it was, I certainly know that it was the right decision, as I wouldn't be without her now. I would just like to say to anyone reading this who is going through a similar time to me, if the services of Macmillan nurses are offered to you, please don't be afraid of accepting it, they will also become a friend as well as being your nurse.

Breast cancer awareness month has now reached an end for another year, the reminders are gone, but for goodness sake don't forget to be aware of your body - only you know what is right or wrong.

I know only too well how frightening it is to make that first appointment with the doctor if something is found that is not quite right, but lumps and bumps do NOT always mean cancer.

So, it's back to the Marsden this week again to see my "new best friends," another tube of wimp cream, another drip, and another hospital special tasteless sandwich. Oh the glamour!

Rhona x

November 10, 2003: *Art of getting on with life when you re dying*

STILL no news on the radiotherapy side, which is not so good. I do wish that doctors wouldn't suggest treatments to raise hopes if there a chance that they can't be carried out for a while, as the waiting is often worse that the treatment itself.

I have however had five tubes of blood taken for genetic testing. I asked about this after I was re-diagnosed, to ensure that screening could be carried out at the earliest stage possible for my children. This blood is now frozen and kept in storage forever at St George's Hospital in London with my consent that DNA can be extracted from it at any time.

It is very reassuring for me to know that, in the future, my blood will be accessible for those who need it, be it my children's children or even further down the family tree.

Francesca, my daughter, has unfortunately shown the first sign of stress in her life, in the form of eczema. I knew it wouldn't be long until something like this happened as she is keeping everything in and pretending that life is normal, in much the same way that my husband David is handling things.

My son Kristopher, however, is rather different and talks to me about everything and asks questions when he feels he needs to know something.

Four years ago, I arranged for both of the children to have counselling, offered to us by St. Nicholas' Hospice in Bury St Edmunds. It was by far one of the best decisions I have ever made as both Kristopher and Francesca came out of this nightmare time as very well adjusted little people.

As soon as our life tumbled upside down again in June, I phoned the hospice up to ask for further counselling. This time, only Kristopher would accept help. It is very worrying as a mum to watch your daughter suffer in silence, knowing that her little heart is breaking by refusing to come to terms with what is happening in the big world.

I do know she has much support from her teachers and headmaster at school and is well looked after during school hours. When I have my daily nap I can do so knowing she is happy and no doubt dreaming of meeting pop idol Justin Timberlake along with her best friend Rosie.

I have always been an outgoing person with quite a silly sense of humour but I have been told by my friends, and have noticed myself, that over the last four months I have changed. I can only describe it as being on a huge adrenaline flow (I do admit to still having very off days. David thinks the best way of dealing with this is to ignore me. How many wives out there get

6

the same treatment? Haven't our husbands worked out yet that we don't want to be ignored, we just want CHOCOLATE!).

Many people have asked me how I keep going knowing that I am dying. The answer is very simple really. I just do.

I have a very close friend who was diagnosed with multiple sclerosis in her early 30s and has now lived with this debilitating disease for more than four years. Although I know that she too has very low days and can't get through a day without her need for sleep, she, like me, has seen a change in her sense of humour. Always a true English rose and very quiet before her life changed, she now sees the funny side of the direction our lives have taken.

We go out often on our "ladies who lunch" days and we just laugh for the whole time. Neither of us are exactly good at walking nowadays and we most definitely do not even have a goldfish memory between us. If you see two blondes trying to cross a road playing drunk, please do not beep your horn as it will only be us enjoying the good part of our lives - without the alcohol.

I have just had a card from my doctor offering me the flu jab (another nasty needle..lovely!). It says this is given to the elderly or at-risk patients. As I feel perfectly well and look quite normal, they have obviously decided that being 42 years, 10 months and 30 days old, I am classified as elderly!

Rhona x

November 17, 2003: *Bad week that left me black and very blue*

EVEN those perched high on the "adrenaline tree" can fall and unfortunately this is what has happened to me during the last week. Thankfully I am coming out of it now, but I have just had the worst week I can ever remember in my life. It is just a shame that very purple eyes aren't in fashion right now because that is how mine have looked for a few days!

It started off when I had to go back to the hospital last week for another drip. Unfortunately after four hours the various chemo nurses (they all had a go!) were still unable to find a decent vein which would be strong enough to take the drip.

Even my last good vein managed to burst so I now have a beautiful multi-coloured black and blue arm and hand (aren't I colourful this week?) but in the end they managed to get the cannula into my wrist by my bone...very painful.

I have however been told that should I need further chemo, which has to be administered intravenously, then the only option for me is have a "pick" line inserted under my skin in my chest which is connected to a vein. Needless to say this is very much frightening me for many reasons, as it would always be a constant reminder of my illness, fear of infection, and of course the surgery to have it inserted in the first place, but in all honesty it looks like this could be my only choice from now on.

By this time I was really feeling unwell, but the day just got worse. When I asked if my results had come back to see if I had the HER2 hormone, I was told that they were still waiting but it was hoped that I hadn't as it would mean that I would then have a very aggressive form of cancer.

So I am now in the situation of do I want this hormone or not? What great choices I have been given!

The end of the day gave me the worst news. I was asked if I wanted to be tested for the BRCA1 and BRCA2 gene. If I tested positive it could mean that prostate cancer might raise its ugly head in years to come with my son. I have obviously agreed to this testing so that along with my daughter, screening can commence at a very early age for both of them. The decision will, of course, have to be theirs as once screening begins for them I have been told by the genetic nurses that they will then have huge problems getting insurance, so right now I am feeling one very guilty mum, and that is not a good feeling to have.

Every mum has proud moments with her children, it starts from the moment that they are born really and never seems to end, so there have been many times when I have been there in various situations with that emotional feeling and the biggest inside smile knowing that I am Kristopher's and Francesca's mum!

The last few months my children have given me two of my proudest days. Francesca was first when she decided she wanted to run in the "Race for Life". It was one of the hottest days we had in the summer. I expected her to walk it as she had not trained in any way for this race, so I sent her off with her pink celebration card pinned on to her back which she had writ-

'My children have given me two of my proudest days'

ten on "For my mummy" and a two-litre bottle of water! Thirty-four minutes later this little girl came running past, face bright red and a full bottle of water, but with a huge smile on her face. When I finally found her in the crowd she said: "I did this for you mummy." What a moment, all I can say is I'm glad I had a tissue!

My second proud moment was on Remembrance Sunday, when I watched my son march with the cadets from RAF Wattisham. It broke my heart knowing that I will never see him in the career of his dreams, which is to be in the RAF. He is so determined to do this, I am sure his dreams will come true one day.

The day was made even more special when Kristopher chose to wear my late dad's black tie, even though he had to have his tie retied for him by his CO, we both knew that his "Gramps" would have been a very proud man.

Well, now it's time to forget what has gone on in the past few days and start to climb that tree again, so I'm off to try to find a fancy dress outfit for Francesca as she is going to a party this week. She has decided to go as a fairy, which is quite funny really, as I have decided to return as a fairy - both good and bad!

The good side of me will be for my family and friends, and the bad..well you'd better beware. Hint, hint - this is going out to my old domestic science teacher, as I do think you ought to know that I will never forgive you for dropping my chocolate cake out of its tin!

Rhona x

November 24, 2003: *What a shock when reality finally kicks in*

GUESS what? I won't be needing that colourful wheelchair after all in Australia as I have started my course of radiotherapy and soon I will have finished it. It all happened very quickly, in the end. I got a letter on Monday, was up to the Marsden on Tuesday, had the tattoos put in place on Wednesday (to pinpoint where the rays will enter), and then the treatment started on Thursday. I have been given a course of five treatments. It doesn't sound like much compared to the full weeks I had last time, but this is a much harsher dosage.

Last time, I was able to drive to Colchester, catch the train at 7am, get on the Circle Line across London, have my treatment, and then do the repeat journey the other way round, arriving home about 4pm to carry on with my day. This time it is all very different. I get picked up by my ambulance car, sleep part of the way, have my five minutes treatment, grab a sandwich from outpatients, sleep most of the way home and then crawl into bed.

When I was treated in 2000, apart from my skin looking sunburnt, I really did not suffer any other side effects from radiotherapy. This time, however, I have severe flu-like symptoms within an hour of my treatment and the worst hangover-type headache you could ever experience.

Before the treatment began, I was finding it very painful to turn my head, but I can thankfully say that it is now much easier to do this, so I think it is working.

A consent form has to be signed before treatment commences, which was not unexpected. What I didn't expect to see were the words "palliative care" and "symptom control" written on the form.

I wasn't sitting down, so the shock of this made me feel quite sick. I obviously became pale as the doctor pulled a chair up for me to sit down. I know that this may sound a bit of silly thing to feel, but to actually see this in black and white and know that, this time, a cure is not an option for me is very frightening. Although 99.9% of me has accepted that I am dying, the other 0.1%, was clinging on to the hope that my diagnosis was wrong. When I saw those words, the true reality hit me that this last tiny percentage had finally

been swallowed up by something bigger.

Of course major disasters don't often just happen once - just as I was coming to terms with my new care package, disaster number two occurred...my mobile phone broke!

For those of you who don't know me, I'm not exactly a quiet person. In fact, I would have to admit that talking is my main hobby.

When I was told that I would not be able to speak after my radiotherapy due to my throat being burnt it was like I had been given a death sentence (oops, slip of the tongue!).

The next best thing for me was text messaging but with my phone having given up the ghost, I just didn't know how I would survive. David thought he had saved the day by offering me his phone but if you could see his phone you would understand I could not accept - honestly, doesn't he realise that I have standards to uphold? Francesca, luckily has lent me her phone now until I sort a new one out. It certainly looks good, it's just a shame it's all too technical for me. I would like to apologise to all those friends who get the same message from me four times over and to say I don't really mean to hang up on you when you call - it is all too complicated for this 42-year-old.

I am feeling very tired now, with being on chemo and radiotherapy, but there has been a bonus for me with having to travel up every day to London. Just five minutes along from the hospital is King's Road - sorry David, but I'm sure deep down you really do understand that we actually do need all those items from Habitat and Heals and the rest!

I have many things that I want to do before my "finale" arrives. I know that many things on my wish list won't ever happen but I'm determined to fit in as many as I can.

This weekend, David and I are off to Bath. We always try to have one weekend away around this time of year without the children, so as Bath is on my list, we are off on Friday.

The children are staying with some friends in Enfield, Lily (our Westie) is having a "sleepover" at David's mum's home and I am off to be wined and dined by my husband. I am back for my drip on Thursday, so it will be so lovely to have this to look forward to after another colourful session at the day unit.

Rhona x

December 1, 2003: *I hope my story will be helpful to others*

JUST when I thought I had escaped the full side-effects from my radiotherapy, it kicked in on Sunday with a huge "ouch".

It has since got even worse. I must admit I am not feeling on top form at the moment. I was told that my throat would be burned - what I wasn't told was that it would also burn my gums, teeth, glands and mouth. I'm not sure if it feels like I've had liposuction that has gone very wrong or have had my mouth wide open in direct sunlight for a week. When I try to eat or drink it is like taking a shower after a full day in the sun without enough sunscreen on. It would unfortunately seem that I have at least a week before this stinging pain starts to ease - David should make the most of the quiet life!

As you know, I have been organising my funeral, and apart from deciding on a burial plot at the church and what I am going to wear (I feel a new dress coming on!) I recently chose my coffin to get me that one step closer to having the full day planned.

I am lucky in that I know Lavenham's funeral director David Deacon quite well from my days when I owned a flower shop in the village and used to arrange all the requested funeral tributes. I asked a friend to go along with me as I knew that she would stay strong for me and help me make the right choice.

David was fantastic handling my request, as it would seem that it is something that doesn't often happen, which surprised me. There was some laughing and joking along with the seriousness of what I was to do.

I knew what I wanted, so it took a little while to finally find it - and then there it was, my "bed" for the next life. After a few phone calls, David managed to carry out all my requirements to allow me to have the exact style, colour and lining that I wanted. The only thing we couldn't quite decide on was the date, but at least I know that when the time does come it will all be there in his diary.

I hope that both my friend and David will have a laugh when they remember the jokes made on that day.

I hope everyone who reads my column realises why I write it every week. I do it for two reasons - to try to maintain awareness of breast cancer and to make people aware that if you have been diagnosed with cancer it doesn't necessarily mean an immediate death sentence.

There can be a life with cancer.

Unfortunately, once you become a cancer patient, it does mean that cancer lives with you. With the help of friends, family and a positive mind, however, life can continue. Of course, there will be many bad days as well as good, but you are still here, and that's the main thing.

When I was first diagnosed, my life did seem to end for a few days. It was my children that made me get up and fight the illness, but I can understand only too well for

10

those who feel they don't have a reason to live, how easy it all would be to give up. I even remember telling Claire, Francesca's godmother, that when it came to the time when things got very bad, how I would arrange for the children to go to a friend's for the day and then I would end my life. Four years on, I know that everything I said then was just the fear talking - I would never consider that to be an option for me now.

As each day goes by I find myself a stronger person than I was the day before.

'As each day goes by I find myself stronger than the day before'

There are often tears, nearly always over something the children have said or done, and when I think of their future I always feel my emotions rising. It is strange really, that life goes on for people like me just in the same way that it might for those grieving. Although we all may look brave on the outside it doesn't mean that we are all not crying on the inside for what might have been.

I have been asked to do an "awareness" documentary for television. They will follow me through the good and bad days ... even film me on a "lunch day". I will write more about this next week, but I feel extremely privileged to have been asked to do this as I hope this will be the true-fact programme of living with cancer which I wanted to watch four years ago, but unfortunately, wasn't available.

I want my story to help those who need to know more, but are unable to find out what life with primary, followed by secondary, cancer is really like.

This, I hope, will give them answers.

Rhona x

December 8, 2003: *Brought down to earth with a crash*

The caption under my photo in the EADT last week said "Bound for Bath" but sadly the wonderful weekend we had planned didn't happen. Instead it was "Bound for Bed" in a morphine haze for yours truly.

I had written how I had woken up with a huge "ouch" when the side-effects of my radiotherapy had hit in, but I didn't quite expect what was to follow.

I am very cross with myself that I didn't ask more about the after-effects. I accepted that I could lose my voice, have a sore throat, and maybe a slight cough, but what I wasn't told was that words would not be able to describe how painful it would be.

My throat actually closed up, blood blisters and sores covered the inside of my mouth, my tongue merged with my gums and the pain in my head and ears was at screaming pitch.

As I write this, I have not eaten for 11 days and have lost 9lb in weight. Drinking sips of liquid is still causing me a major problem, but at least I have now started to cope without the morphine.

I was supposed to have it every four hours but needed it every two - it had to be syringed into my mouth as I was unable to take it from a spoon.

All of this would have been easier to accept if this harsh treatment was the means to a cure. As it is classified as "symptom control" with no guarantee it will work, I am annoyed that over two weeks of good quality life have been taken away from me. That is something I can no longer afford to happen in what is left of my new, shortened, life.

I was meant to have another "blast" next week but I am afraid to say that I have decided against this and any further treatment - unless the side-effects are low enough for me to keep my everyday life going just how I want it.

When things go wrong, everything seems to conspire to plunge you into an all-time low, so I suppose events of last week should not have been any great surprise.

Just when I was feeling at my absolute worst, an hour into our journey to the Marsden (to have my drip), in rush-hour traffic, we had a car crash. Our ambulance car driver, who we have got to know very well, had a dreadful ordeal. Luckily for all of us, we didn't have too many bumps or injuries, but the car was quite a wreck.

As all of the drivers do this wonderful service on a voluntary basis, it seemed to me even more distressful that something so awful should happen to someone who had given up their own time to help others.

Looking back now I think I hit a huge hysterical moment, just after the crash, when I was sitting in the car on the outside lane quite shaken and also feeling extremely sick (all the men involved were standing outside). Ian, our driver, jumped into the car saying that we were on fire. Instead of panicking I remained seated and thought "Oh great, I have survived cancer all this time and now I'm going to die in a fire."

But did I make a move out of that car? Oh no, I stayed right where I was, trying to look as serene as possible - just how daft was that?

Anyway, as you can gather, the car did not catch fire and I remain in this world for a little longer. When we finally reached the hospital, I found miracles do happen as my cannula found its way into a vein first time. That was quickly followed by some bad news (just for a change!).

The HER2 positive hormone that I so desperately wanted so I could be given the new wonder drug Herceptin was not present in my blood sample. That means that, unfortunately, I will not be one of the lucky people to trial the drug.

A 23-year-old girl was sitting next to me having the Herceptin injection as I had just been given this news and I felt a strange sort of jealousy run through me. It is a terrible thing for me to admit to, but I thought why should she have it and not me? After all, she wasn't a mother who wanted more than anything to watch her children grow up.

Then, the true reality of her situation finally hit me - what right did I have to be jealous of her? How dare I feel this animosity towards her? After all, I have had the wonderful experience of being a wife and a mother of two.

The fact that she was being given this drug meant that she had the worst form of aggressive cancer possible, so she would most likely never have those extra 20 years which I have had. I don't have any regrets in my life and have been able to do most things I have wanted to do, but this beautiful young girl will never have that chance to fulfil her life with all her fantasies and ambitions.

As I said, we never made Bath, but it will remain on my list of somewhere that I will visit before I join my dad, who is waiting for me with a nice full glass of red wine!!

I briefly mentioned last week that I have been asked by Anglia Television to work on a documentary with them about living with cancer and my determination to openly talk about this disease. Two wonderful people, Natalie and Tony, have been given the difficult job of working with me. I hope that together we can do what I have always looked for but never found - a story of a normal, everyday person living with cancer, showing all the good, the bad, and the emotions that go with it.

I have so far spent three days with these two lovely people, who I now feel I have known all my life, trying to show how life really is for the high percentage of us who have to come to terms with living with this often killer disease.

I am not doing this for my 15 minutes of fame, but for those of you, who like me, four years ago, are scared of the unknown and need true answers.

Well, its back to the life of Lucozade and Build-up for me, until I can manage to swallow properly again!

Rhona x

December, 15, 2003: *Sometimes it s hard to hold back the tears*

AT last...I can talk again!! Although I still have some pain in my mouth, I am very much back to normal (which is surprising, really, as I have never been normal before!)

Last Monday, I phoned my Macmillan nurse as I did not seem to be getting any pain relief from the medication I was on and was still finding it difficult to swallow anything which wasn't soft.

Once again she knew exactly what I needed, phoned around until she got a positive answer, and the following day I was on a new medicine. Within 24 hours the pain started to ease in my throat; by the end of the week I had managed to put on two pounds in weight, then on Sunday had a wonderful roast dinner cooked to perfection by my friend Julia.

This whole ordeal has been something which I won't forget in a hurry, and has made the whole cancer diagnosis very real. Francesca, unfortunately, is very low right now so it was not a surprise when she went down with the latest flu which seems to be hitting young people. As this happened at the same time as my radiotherapy side-effects, some days she spent much of her day in bed with me.

I would often wake up to find her looking at me, and of course it didn't need too much working out as to what was going through her mind. I found all of this deep thinking of hers quite a strain on me as I wanted to cry when I looked at her beautiful but sad eyes. But of course, I couldn't let her see my tears.

I admit I do cry often but try not to in front of the children, as I know that would upset them even more. So the brave, smiley face, which I try to manage when those tears are close, had to make its appearance during those days.

I obviously looked quite close to departing at one stage, because she woke me up to ask me if I wanted Lily (our Westie) at my funeral! This is one of the few arrangements that I haven't worked out for the day in question, but I have now decided I would like, if possible, our naughty little puppy there as she will bring the comfort needed by my gorgeous little girl.

Just before I became ill, I did some photographs for a new company called "Wim Wham Fashions" for their forthcoming catalogue and website. I have always complained about how there is just nothing out there for women like me who have had mastectomies and reconstructive surgery, and then at last there is, the chance to feel glamorous again in beautifully designed and outstanding nightwear, tops and bustiers.

I and another girl, who has also under-

13

gone surgery, had a very special day, being pampered before the 'shoot' by a professional lady who did our hair and make-up, followed by glasses of champagne, salmon and strawberries!

Many photos were taken in all sorts of outfits and poses, so it will be all very exciting to see the finished website and brochure. I would just like to say to those who are maybe in a similar position to me and would like to feel very feminine again, please do contact Carol on 01787 278094 for details, as this is definitely a company for us 'GIRLS'!

I have found Christmas very difficult to handle this year. As I have wandered around the shops, I feel myself listening to all the carols being played and for the first time have found it all very sad. The words seem to be rather poignant, and I keep going back to the same thought of "will I be here for next Christmas?"

I think deep down I probably know the answer to this question but am scared of acknowledging it to myself, as I can't bear the thought of my children without me at Christmas.

All of this sadness I am experiencing now has been deepened by the recent news that I cannot have the drug Herceptin. This, I believe, was my last big chance of lengthening my life, and the fact that I now can't have it is devastating to me. Maybe, though, I should be relieved as all the cancer drugs which I have been on have aged me.

As you read this, David and I will be in the middle of a huge row as we put the last few items into our suitcases. As usual, no doubt, David will be sitting on the cases as we try to get them shut, with him telling me that I really don't need that fifth pair of shoes. But of course I do; even if I don't actually wear them I will have them with me...just in case!

'Will I be here for next Christmas?'

Christmas for the four of us this year will be very different to all the others, but one that will be very special. I'm really not filled with the Christmas spirit as I write this and maybe will find that we really won't feel very festive this year. But even if it doesn't, we will be together as a family, enjoying a much-deserved but also a special holiday that will never be forgotten.

My best friend Louise and her family are coming down for the weekend and on the Sunday I am having an open house for friends to come for mulled wine and nibbles, so it will be a lovely start to our trip to Oz.

Rhona x

January 5, 2004: *When I set alarm bells ringing in LA*

G'day...can you guess who it is yet? Obviously the sun has gone to my head and I am now talking like Rolf Harris.

Well, we are in paradise, although I am finding it just too hot. We have had our time in Brisbane and are just about to leave Noosa, Queensland, to fly to Heron Island on the Great Barrier Reef for Christmas. I know for certain that it will be a very quiet celebration as Down Under is nothing like Christmas at home. None of the shops are decorated and there doesn't seem to be the annual rush to buy last-minute presents! I think they have the right idea here - it is so laid back, instead of all the stress and panic we all seem to get into before the big day.

I haven't had too many problems with my health so far, although the 33-hour flight here did leave me so tired that I slept for 20 hours after arriving in Brisbane. My feet had swelled so much by the end of the flight I saw a lot of people looking at them - mind you I was in a wheelchair!

We have been here now almost a week and my feet still don't feel right but then neither does my stomach, with all the drugs, and my liver is now so swollen I really don't feel comfortable.

Even with all that, we are all very lucky to be here as six months ago it didn't seem likely I would make another Christmas, never mind make it to the other side of the world.

The only major problem we have had with our journey was in Los Angeles. Unfortunately, my recent radiotherapy was still in my body so I set off alarm bells going through Customs. Having just got off a 12-hour flight, I wasn't in the mood for what was to happen next.

I was made to take my shoes off and go through the scanner again. As the alarm went off for a second time, I was then made to stand in front of everyone on a special mat and remove many items of my clothing. I tried to explain about my treatment but they had, at that stage, decided I was a criminal and proceeded to humiliate me. Even when they reduced me to tears they still did not show any compassion.

We finish up in LA before our return journey so I am not looking forward to clearing Customs again.

I hope everyone had a great Christmas. We will be in Sydney for New Year celebration and I am meeting up with a friend I haven't seen for 14 years. We have arranged to spend the evening with Diane and her family and soak up every minute of the atmosphere.

I will end this postcard home by wishing everyone at home a very happy and healthy New Year...

Hi from Sydney. Hope everyone had a great Christmas and that Santa brought you all that was wished for!!

We are now on stage three of our holiday and it is all going by very fast. Our Christmas on the Great Barrier Reef was very different but one that none of us will ever forget. Santa arrived by helicopter and with sunglasses on! Each child on the island received a present and old girls like me got to look. Lunch was a huge buffet with seafood in a quantity I have never seen before. The children had brought their stockings so they woke up to find lots of little Aussie goodies in them. The afternoon was spent relaxing by the pool...how civilized!

On Christmas night we were taken turtle watching, which had to be the most wonderful piece of nature I have ever experienced. As we did not get back until 1am, however, I paid the price on Boxing Day.

This was the day on which I thought I would need a drip as soon as I reached Sydney as I was in so much pain. With this, of course, came the depression and the thought of how likely it was that this would be our last holiday. I watched David and the children throughout the day and tried to imagine their lives without me.

David is such a good dad. I know that both K & F will be so well cared for and loved by him and that he will try to replace a mum's love as much as possible.

As each day ends it frightens me that we will be returning to our real life once again. Over here I can forget what is going on but as soon as that BA jumbo hits the tarmac at Heathrow then I will once again become the terminally ill cancer patient. I will have missed two drips by then so I expect I will be in a lot of pain. Until then though it is back to our fantasy world.

As I write this I am looking forward to seeing in the New Year tomorrow night at the Sydney Harbour Bridge with a million other people. I am meeting a very good friend tomorrow at Manly and we are having a champagne dinner before the fireworks begin.

Although I haven't seen Diane for many years it will also be a sad time for us as we both know this will be the last time we will ever meet up. I don't know how either of us will say goodbye but I'm sure there will be a few tears.

We will continue until the end of the week being true tourists before flying to Hawaii and then finish off by probably once again setting off alarm bells in LA airport...

But, until I write again, HAPPY NEW YEAR TO ALL OF YOU!!

Rhona x

January 12, 2004: *Scaling new heights on my fabulous trip Down Under*

HI from Los Angeles. Unfortunately we are at the end of our wonderful trip now.

The big news from me is I CLIMBED THE SYDNEY HARBOUR BRIDGE!!

This was something which six months ago I thought was unreachable for me, but on Saturday, January 3 at 5am, I started the climb and completed the 1400 steps and stood at the top of that bridge and watched the sun rise over Sydney.

I have the photos taken by our guide so hopefully I will be able to include one in my diary when I get back home.

New Year's Eve in Sydney was something different - would you believe that I bumped into someone I know from home?! More details of the holiday will follow.

We will soon be on our way back home and with that the thought of it now being 2004 I am worried that this could be my final year.

It always seemed so far away thinking that it could all happen next year but now that we have reached 2004 I am getting frightened.

I am trying to be as positive as possible about the return but it is not as easy as I would hope.

As much as I don't want this all to end, however, I feel that now is the right time to go home as I am getting very tired and am feeling the effects of having missed two drips. But I am waiting for all our photos to arrive and relive the memories!

Rhona x

January 19, 2004: *Normality starts to kick in*

G'DAY, Aloha and Hi...How clever am I to have learned all these greetings?!

Well I'm sorry to say the big Oz adventure is all over now and normality is starting to kick in for all of us.

As I write this, however, we are all still waking up at midnight, eating cereal at 4am and watching DVDs at 5am. We still have the Christmas tree and cards up - including those from my birthday in early December - unpacked suitcases in each room, washing still packed tightly in hotel laundry bags and, in all honesty, we feel pretty rough.

The whole trip seemed to flash past very quickly but, at the same time, it seems a very long time ago that we started out on that 33-hour journey. We were adamant that it should be a holiday of a lifetime.

In the past we have gone away and foolishly spent too much time on beaches and just generally chilling out but this time we could not afford to do that - I simply don't have the time.

Each day we ventured into something new and, apart from being by the pool for a few hours after Christmas lunch, we lived each waking hour to the full.

Admittedly, in the last few days, I started to get very tired, so really for me, the holiday was about the right length. That doesn't stop me from wishing that I was still living the beautiful life Down Under.

I was extremely lucky with my health. I had expected to go into hospital in Sydney for a bone-drip, but fortunately I think someone must have been watching over me. Apart from Boxing Day, I did not suffer from a great deal of pain.

The news, however, is not all wonderful. I will know more over the coming weeks when I head back to the Marsden for scans but my cough is now creeping back and I am finding that by the time I have climbed the stairs I am starting to wheeze. Also, my liver is starting to cause some discomfort and is now beginning to look quite enlarged and my tummy is quite swollen. I have been waiting for someone to ask me when I'm due.

I had packed summer clothes, many of which I hadn't worn for a few months, so was distressed when they wouldn't fit. I have always been quite tiny so this extra stone in weight is not to my liking at all!

However, this didn't spoil the main highlight of the trip for me - climbing the Sydney Harbour Bridge.

Before starting, everyone is breathalysed, including the children, and all medical conditions had to be declared. I was scared they wouldn't let me climb - especially with my eyesight - so I played down my condition somewhat.

Halfway up, however, I had the worst breathing attack I have ever had. Our guide had been told what could happen so was great. I think it was the first time in the last six months that any of us have been really scared - I hated both K & F having to see their mum in so much distress.

I always thought I would be able to hide symptoms in front of the children but suddenly we weren't pretending any more. This was the real thing, and absolutely no amount of acting would soften the situation to avoid upsetting them. Most of the bridge climb steps are vertical but when we came to the end of that particular step my breathing was calmer and I found the rest a lot easier.

'The whole of Sydney stretched out below us'

The sun was just rising as we started. When we reached the top, the whole of Sydney stretched out below us - a fresh, new wonderful morning.

We each had headphones on so that Mike, our leader, could give us facts and information throughout. He was a typical young handsome Aussie surfing dude (If only I had been 20 years younger). He had our group of 12 in stitches with all his jokes. He told us all rugby players refer to the sails of the opera house as "nuns in a scrum." From that height, it was easy to see why. It took us three-and-a-half hours from beginning to end, which included a briefing, climbing into the safety suits and being hooked up to headsets and harnesses. At the start of the climb everyone is clipped on to a continuous wire on handrails at the side of the bridge. These are not unclipped again until the very end, so it is very safe.

Just one word of advice for anyone contemplating climbing the bridge - at the beginning do not look up!!

Now for the facts... The bridge has a sweeping curve 503m long, is 134m high and 49m wide - it is very, very big!

After our absolute delight at having achieved what we had thought was out of the question, we were each presented with a group photo of us all at the top and a cer-

tificate. When the official gave me a silver-framed photograph of the four of us the children couldn't fully understand why I was overcome with emotion.

Over the next few weeks I'll tell you more about the many memories Australia, Hawaii and LA have given us.

One mishap took place, however, during a reef walk on the Great Barrier Reef. I attached our digital camera to my wrist and continued to walk with my hand dangling in the water beside me.

I have broken the camera but neither David nor myself have the nerve to check if I have ruined all the photos on the memory card too. Thankfully, I did take quite a lot of photos with a still camera, so at least we will have something to look back on....

Rhona x

January 26, 2004: *And now for the not-so-good news*

THE saying goes: "All good things must come to an end." Obviously our holiday has, but unfortunately so has the good health I have enjoyed over the past month.

As I write this I have been in bed for four days with a mixture of things. I had a visit to the Marsden last Thursday where I had my long-overdue bone-drip, a check-up and an eye appointment.

Natalie and Tony who are working on the documentary also joined David and myself on this "exciting?" day. I gave my full permission for this to be filmed, but unfortunately the PR for the hospital had different ideas and didn't allow much to be filmed.

This will sound quite funny, but it is MY cancer and not theirs (OOPS back to the playground!) If I don't mind scans etc. being talked about, then I think it should be allowed.

Hardly anything was agreed to, even when I was having the cannula put in (one

of the main things about cancer treatment).

Tony was only allowed to film when I was having my arm cleaned and then afterwards so it will seem that the needle in my vein will have reached there by magic!

The news was good and not so good. The pain which I am experiencing might not be from my liver but instead from my ribs (good because I don't think that my ribs can kill me).

The tumours in my eyes are at present inactive (very, very good news)! But the damage to my eyesight has already been done. My eye specialist, however, was happy to speak to Tony and Natalie about the eye situation and show them the photographs which were taken on the day.

The bad news was that the extensive shaking, which meant I had to spend a day in hospital on the Friday before we went on holiday, could have been a seizure caused by the tumours in my brain. This was not what

18

I wanted to hear. However, I had my drip and, although it does not usually cause any side-effects, this time I have had severe headaches, flu-ish symptoms and more pain than I have ever had before in some of my bones. Whenever I do anything it feels as though all the bones in my hands and arms are broken. I can feel quite close to tears with the pain.

I am also suffering the worst fatigue I can remember. I have not been out of bed for more than five minutes when I have to get back in because I am so breathless. It is even more tiring when I try to calm my breathing down. The rib/liver pain has also worsened and even though I just want to sleep all the time I'm finding it hard to find a comfortable position so that I do not feel the burning pain.

Of course, much of the tiredness has probably been as a direct result of having put so much energy into Australia and not letting myself have too much time off. The lack of sunshine doesn't help either. We all know how the sun can bring out the best in us.

The fact that the excitement of Oz is long gone is also a factor. I am at the hospital twice next week for scans. Why they both can't be arranged for the same day is beyond me. But what has my health, going up and down to London on separate days, or the money spent on transport got to do with me?

And what of the fact that I hate injections so much it would be much kinder for me to have one cannula instead of two different needles. But hey, that's the life of a cancer patient!

The good news is that at last we have managed to download all the photographs from our broken digital camera and we can now bore all our friends. Just you dare go to sleep!

Since coming home I have received so many lovely letters of support. Thank you all so much. I will always be a complete stranger to all of you, so it is very emotional knowing that so many of you are thinking of us and saying prayers for my family. Every letter and card will be kept for my children to read in years to come. I know that they, too, will feel the same emotion that I am feeling that so many people can take time out of their busy lives to sit down and write to someone who they will never know. Thank you again.

In turn, I hope that I am also helping other families who are going through a similar situation to us. By sharing our experiences, I hope they will not feel they have to suffer alone and will see how having cancer can be a life of many ups and downs.

My memories of Down Under will continue next week but in the meantime I would like to share with you something I read while on holiday.

It made me stop and think because I knew how true it was. Some of you may have read this before but for those of you who haven't, I hope it will mean as much to you as it does me. "HAPPINESS IS A JOURNEY, NOT A DESTINATION."

For a long time it seemed to me that life was about to begin - real life, but there was always some obstacle in the way, something to get through first, some unfinished business, time to be served, a debt to be paid.

'Thank you all so much for your prayers'

19

At last it has dawned on me that these obstacles were my life. This perspective has helped me to see that there is no way to happiness. Happiness is the way, so treasure every moment you have and remember that time waits for no one.

Rhona x

February 2, 2004: *A week of highs and lows*

IT has been an all sorts of a week here. There has been laughter, tears, silliness, enjoyment, sickness and noisy opinions. But right at the moment as I write, there is snow!

I was getting very disappointed as time was getting on and we hadn't got the forecasted blizzards. I have always loved snow but this time, for obvious reasons, I am very excited and determined to enjoy every minute of it.

I need to get up quite a lot during the night, so have spent the last few looking out of the window at all hours hoping to see the first flakes. At last, this morning, there it was. Both of the children's schools are closed so they too are making the most of it, with K doing the masculine thing of throwing snowballs, while F is out using her artistic talents crafting a snowman!

Me, well I'm just going to watch it through the window in front of a log fire, happy inside that I can watch the beauty of another season.

I have been feeling very nauseous and tired over the past few days. I hate this feeling of not being in control. I'm back on the anti-sickness tablets. I'm not sure what the cause is. Of course my mind works overtime on occasions like this - it is hard for me to think that it might just be one of the many bugs doing their rounds at this time of year. I naturally believe it is my liver, after all, it is one of the symptoms.

Itching of the skin is strangely another one and I certainly have that. Thankfully, I have not yet turned yellow - when that happens, I know I am definitely in trouble. The results of my scans should be known this Thursday. Once again I will ask them for a prognosis but, no doubt, once again I will leave not knowing how much time I have left to play with.

My friend Laini and I went to see the film *Love Actually* last week. We've wanted to see it for ages as everyone told us how good it was. We had not quite reckoned on some of the content, which proved a little too close to home. The funeral of a mum with a young son was rather poignant and I could feel my

> 'I could feel my eyes starting to fill up'

eyes starting to sting and fill up. The worst was still to come when Eva Cassidy's version of *Songbird* was played...this is the song I have chosen to accompany my coffin as it is carried out of the church. A feeling of sickness ran through me; *Songbird* is one of her less played songs and although I play it at home, I never imagined I would hear it watching a comedy.

David and I went to York last weekend to spent some lovely time with my friends John and Elizabeth, who I have known since I was a child. They always spoil me - they

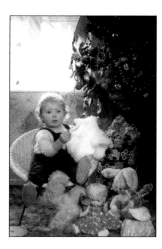

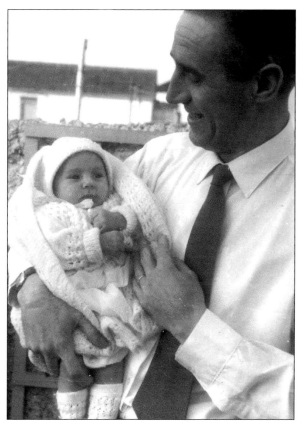

CHRISTMAS MAGIC: Rhona's first Christmas, above, and second, below, shared with a friendly snowman

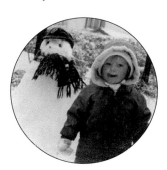

SAFE IN DADDY'S ARMS: Baby Rhona, with dad John

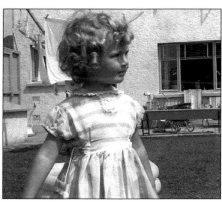

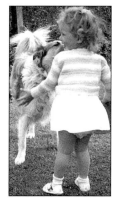

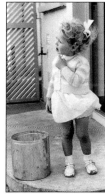

EARLY DAYS: Curly-haired Rhona finds her feet at her home in Northern Ireland

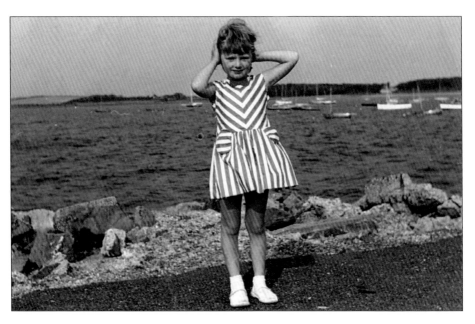

FASHION SENSE: Rhona aged about six, and a little stripey number hints at things to come

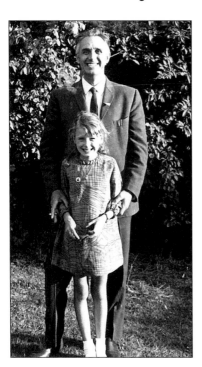

FATHER'S PRIDE: Rhona with her dad, left, aged eight in July, 1969, and, right, moving into woman-hood and looking stunning in green

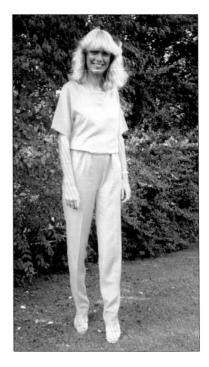

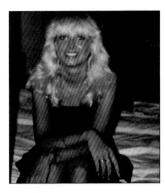

SWEET SIXTEEN: Rhona on holiday in her teens and, below, at 23 as a fondness for a tipple becomes evident

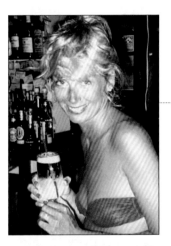

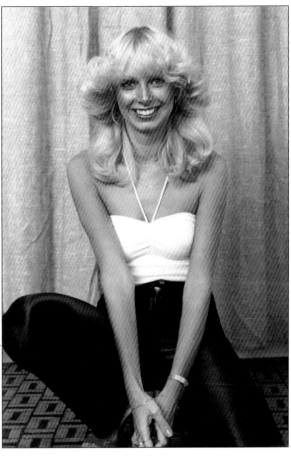

GLAMOUR GIRL: Rhona as a very striking 17-year-old

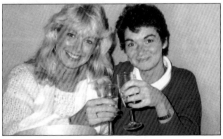

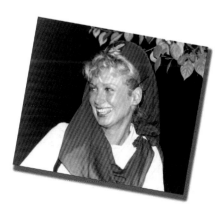

FUN-LOVING: Rhona shares some champers with her friend Louise and, right, looks stylish in her role as a Gulf Air stewardess. In both photographs Rhona is aged 23

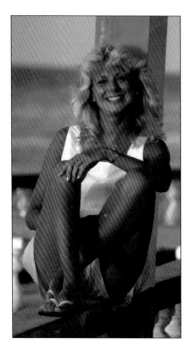

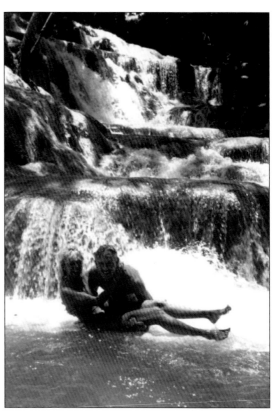

LOVE BLOSSOMS: Right, **Rhona and David embrace in a waterfall in Jamaica in 1985.** Above, **the first photograph David ever took of his wife-to-be, also in Jamaica, 1985**

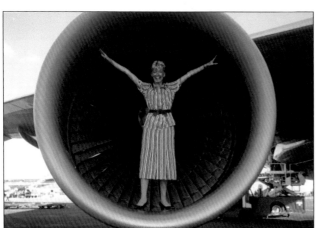

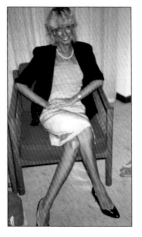

GLOBE-TROTTER: Rhona stands in one of the engines of a 747 airliner in Mauritius during her time as a British Airways stewardess and, right, **relaxing in Raffles Hotel, Singapore**

are as close to family as you can get. I usually go up to York by myself so have done all the touristy things before but as this was David's first visit we revisited the sights together.

One of the main highlights for David was definitely our visit to the Minster. There was a true sense of calm and serenity and it seemed fitting that I should have a candle lit for me but I was also very surprised as David has never done this before.

That made my eyes prickle but it was when Elizabeth put my name forward to be included in the daily prayers that the tears started to roll. I didn't want any of them to see, so was relieved when my mobile went off (I know that this should have been switched off but I'm afraid my memory is not so good any more!).

I had chosen carefully what clothing (or rather picked out that which actually still fitted me) to wear for the meal in the evening so it was with much laughter that David came back from the car with two boots - both for my left foot. Another reminder that my mind does not work properly anymore!

I have always tried to kept my fear of needles away from K and F, but obviously not well enough. I watched my son suffer over the thought of his BCG which he had to have at the beginning of the week. For days before he was very tearful and scared - he didn't sleep the night before, just as I don't before my needles.

On the day, I would not leave the house as I expected the school to ring. Thankfully they didn't but when he returned home he told me in exact detail of how it had affected him.

If I hadn't been watching him speak I would have sworn that it was me explaining how I feel having injections. What have I done , passing a fear like this on to my son?

One of the main reasons we moved here many years ago was the fact that our house looks out over farmland. It has been beautiful for me to lie in bed on my very unwell days, with the window open listening to the birds singing. It was very distressing, therefore, to find out on arriving home from Australia, that the farmer who owns the land wants to sell it for lorry parking, boat building and a car park!

Not only will he devalue our homes damaging our children's inheritance, interfere with all the wildlife that has made its home on his farm, but most of all, he will deprive us of our peace (to say nothing of the light pollution).

It seems very unfair that a residential estate can suddenly have HGV lorries allowed, driving through our roads and working right on the edge of our gardens.

There will be a time when my bedroom will become my solace. Although I will be under sedation to take the pain away I fear that, if this goes ahead, I will be living the last of my life not in the calm and peaceful surroundings of my home, but in a noisy, smelly industrial estate...something more to look forward to.

Our holiday photos have now returned and with them the longing to go back. This week's memory is that of our visit to the Australian Zoo. Steve Irwin the crocodile hunter wasn't there that day as his baby son had just arrived into the world.

I have been to many zoos over the years since having children but this was the best by far. Francesca's dream of holding a koala came true and K got to hold both a python and an alligator. Many animals were allowed to roam freely through this magnificent and vast open parkland.

We are lucky to have all of this on video, so that we will be able to look back on visiting what we would all call the best zoo ever!

Rhona x

February 9, 2004: *Losing control of my life is so scary*

As dictated by Rhona from her bed in the Royal Marsden Hospital, Fulham Road, London.

I previously wrote about how I had two scans on two different days - an arrangement which didn't seem at all logical.

This time, I was determined to have things my way. The Marsden granted me my wish.

Back in hospital for CT and bone scans, I didn't feel too happy about any of it, right from the moment of waking up, but was unsure why. Isn't instinct an amazing thing?

As they had to inject two dyes, for contrast, I opted for a cannula, only to discover that my only good vein was in my thumb. The pain of this was sickening and stayed with me throughout the day. A large amount of dye was needed for the CT, which resulted in my wrist becoming very swollen, black and sore.

We had just left the Marsden to begin our journey home when my mobile phone rang. It was a doctor telling me I had an abnormal amount of fluid around my heart, meaning I now had a life-threatening condition and should be admitted into hospital straight away.

We compromised and agreed I could go in on Saturday but she made me promise to do nothing until then. I would need surgery at the Royal Brompton Hospital to correct this but, until then, I would be a guest of the Marsden.

The hours in between have been spent under a haze of swollen, tearful eyes and thoughts of how I am supposed to give in to now letting my life go.

Apart from the breathlessness, which had started to creep in after Australia, with intermittent pain, I actually didn't feel like a dying woman. I had thought that, with cancer, the time would come when things got so bad that letting go would feel like the right thing to do.

Here I was, not ready to let go and yet the decision was starting to be made for me.

Both K and F behaved in different ways, with David being rather quiet. Scared really doesn't sum up how I felt leaving home. My little Lily (my Westie) knew something was going on. It didn't help much that she cuddled into me when I said goodbye.

I left home not feeling like a cancer patient but now, five days later, I have achieved the hospital greyness, along with the black circles under my eyes from lack of sleep.

There is now little resemblance to the person who had just got back from holiday.

Blood has been taken; chest X-ray, ECG and an ultrasound have been carried out.

It seems I have just under one litre of fluid around my heart, with the wall in danger of collapsing under the pressure, and yet my operation seems to be postponed each day. It would seem that even though the two hospitals are only minutes apart, communication between them is almost non-existent.

The operation, which has a very fancy name, has still not been fully explained to me as no one from the Brompton has been available to talk to me. The only thing I know is that a "window" will be cut somewhere around my heart so that the fluid can drain into my stomach. Yet another scar in my chest!

My family and I are becoming more distressed as each day passes. Nothing seems to be moving except for my mind. Although this seemed to be an urgent case on Friday, since arriving things have all been rather laid-back.

I have been told I need to stay under observation and that by staying here I will have priority status for a bed in the

Brompton. The ward I am on now feels like home to me, as this is my third stay.

There is a wide range of ladies; those who have been newly diagnosed and those with secondaries like me, but also those who are on a regime of morphine and constant sleep. I am forever reminded that this will be my life, at some stage. A cancer patient often understands what the last chapter will mean but to have to watch it 24 hours a day is just too close for comfort. It forces you to come to terms with your own mortality and does little to help maintain the positive attitude that we are all told to have.

I watched my mum die a long, painful death and now, almost 30 years later, with all the latest technology, the reality today doesn't seem to have altered much from my memories of that time.

I'm in a hospital miles away from home, frightened and realising that after seven months of terminal cancer I'm getting to the stage of no longer having the control I would like to have over my life.

David and the children stayed over the weekend but are now doing the daily return journey back and forth from Sudbury after school every day. I decided that life should go on as normally as possible for K and F so, much against their wishes, they are at school each day.

There's a packed case in the car, however, so they can come up to stay at short notice when the operation finally takes place.

We rent an apartment, five minutes from the hospital, during times like this.

I have brought the children's memory books into hospital as I felt I should try to complete them now, but in all honesty the tears won't let me see what I'm writing.

Well, fingers crossed, when I write next week's diary I will be back home where I belong, with my family and friends. I can't say I will miss the electric bed, hospital food or lack of television but the manicure and massage I have had will be something I would like to continue back in Waldingfield.

Who would have thought? One month ago, I was climbing Sydney Harbour Bridge and now here I am with a heart that is in danger of giving up.

What a funny old life!

Rhona x

> '*I no longer have the control over my life I would like*'

February 16, 2004: *Recovering in hospital*

RHONA was unable to write her usual column this week as she was recovering from surgery at the Royal Brompton Hospital in London.

Surgeons made an opening (a window) in the fibrous sac surrounding Rhona's heart to allow them to drain off fluid that was preventing the heart from working efficiently. The procedure is called a subxiphoid pericardial window.

Rhona's husband David said the operation had been a success. He said she was very tired but recovering well and very pleased to have been allowed home.

February 23, 2004: *Back home at last, and it feels great*

NORMALLY our annual two-week holiday in the sun always seems to go so quickly.

But my recent 'holiday' in hospital seemed to last an age. Though I did, of course, still manage to come home with all the washing and the peeling skin just like I would normally do.

To my amazement, I also came home with more 'luggage' than I took in. Only I could have two weeks of solid confinement but still manage to shop.

So here I am, at home, with my holdall and two large plastic bags marked "Patient's property"!

But home is where I am now and a place which, in all honesty, I didn't think I would see again.

Where do I start? Well, once again I have been on a road without a light in sight. But once again I have defied the odds and found that sparkling light at the end.

I am in a slightly depressed mood. But is it really surprising? I have a very sore five-inch scar and luminous bruising. I feel tired, have so little colour I feel like a relative of the Grim Reaper and have horrible memories of the surgery.

Then there is my consultant who told me I was only caught just in time. Normally, I can pick myself up quite quickly if I get into a black mood, but this time I think it might take a little longer.

Letters and cards have been coming in from many EADT readers. So, once again, can I say a huge "THANK YOU". It means so much knowing that many thoughts and prayers are with us. People are so unbelievably kind and thoughtful.

So what happened then?

Well, two days after I last wrote, I was on the move to the Brompton, which specialises in heart and lungs. Although it is horrible to be away from home, I have been very fortunate throughout my illness to have been looked after in the top hospitals London has to offer.

My consultant came to see me early on the Friday morning and said he needed to take blood from an artery on my wrist. As you all know I am the greatest wimp in the world with needles so asked to have the "baby magic cream" and if he could come back in an hour.

In hindsight, I find it quite funny giving orders to a top doctor but he dutifully returned with his awful syringe. Even with the cream and the sedative, I can honestly say I have never experienced so much pain from a needle and was very close to passing out. I was told I would be transferred to the Brompton after lunch. But I fell asleep and woke up at 4pm!

I quickly packed all my belongings and was taken the full minute away by ambulance smartly dressed in my night clothes! My initial thoughts of the hospital were of pure hatred. It seemed so old and had a mixed ward. When another doctor came to take even more blood, that was it. I wanted home.

When I arrived, agency nurses were on and I was scared there would be no continuity and no one who would understand my fear of needles. My mood changed into a

> *'I have defied the odds and found that sparkling light'*

slightly childish one as I sulked and sat with fed-up expression on my face.

However, next day things were different. I woke to find that there were wonderful, full-time staff on the ward and breakfast was good. I had visits from the anaesthetist and doctors. I thought I had been on my best behaviour with the doctors but later read in my notes they had described it as a "difficult consultation." Cheek!

The procedure was explained to me and I signed my consent forms. All that was left to do now was wait - until 9am on Monday.

The nursing staff were brilliant. David and the children arrived early on the Saturday with Monopoly.

Throughout the day I had telephone calls from friends but, as the hours passed, my blood pressure rose and I started to feel claustrophobic and anxious.

So, unknown to anyone, I took one of my Lorazepam tablets which I am supposed to have when I have my bone-drips. Very naughty, I know, but it was the only way to get through those long hours.

Sunday brought my friends Anna and Tim who helped take my mind off the following day's ordeal. Some more Lorazepam helped too.

That night saying goodbye to the children was worse than when I had to tell them how ill I was, because I did not think I would see them again.

I knew the risks because I had been told by the doctors how "frail" I was and how, to me, this would be major surgery.

Both K & F wanted to be with me the next morning, but I knew I could not agree to it, so just this once I had to stand my ground and ask them to stay away.

Surprisingly, I had a good night's sleep thanks to the sleeping tablets I was given. I couldn't believe it when I was woken at 6am by a nurse telling me to have a shower and to change into the most wonderful designer hospital gown. Before I knew it I was being collected for theatre. David went with me as far as he could. A quick kiss and he was gone. All I can remember was the coldness of the room and shouting when a cannula was inserted into my hand.

8.45am was the last time I looked at the clock and then, to my absolute delight because it meant I was still alive, it was 4 pm. I was in recovery/intensive care with equipment that belonged in a *Star Wars* film. I was sitting up, with tubes coming from what seemed like every vein in my body. It was then I saw a doctor who explained that both of my lungs had collapsed during surgery and I was going to have to have something known as CPAP - continuous positive airway pressure.

This, he explained, would be the pressure you would feel if you put your head out of a window whilst driving at 100mph. I was to be kept there for at least the next 24 hours as I would have one-to-one nursing.

In between morphine-dazed sleeps, new nursing staff came on for the night, and I was given the gentlest of nurses.

The CPAP was horrendous. I thought that I had to have it on continuously, so only had it removed for a few moments throughout the long night for little sips of water.

It was only the following day, when my surgeon praised me for tolerating it that I heard I could have had some respite for short periods of time. But apparently, by putting up with it, I increased my recovery by 10 times!

When I was woken at 7am for a wash I felt very pleased with myself for coming through this ordeal to be able to tell the story!

The following day I was transferred to the "high-dependency ward". It was in this ward that I spent the night of my dreams with three men! What more can I say? It was due to them that I managed to get home five days early as their manly habits brought me to the conclusion that I needed out of that ward!

Commodes are part of the furniture on HDU and having to listen to running commentary from them each time they went, I knew I had to push myself to extreme measures to ensure escape.

Within a few hours of arriving I was up and walking and made a point of letting the nursing staff know I was mobile. I was elated when I asked if I could move to a normal ward and they said yes!

My rehabilitation came on so much after that day and though I still had to have a drip to boost my potassium levels, many of the tubes started to come out.

At last, on Friday, my blood had reached an acceptable level. I was walking around quite straight, my stitches had been taken out from a larger wound than I had imagined and my eating had returned to normal. So when my consultant did his ward round, I sheepishly asked if I could go home. He agreed but on the understanding that I was to take it easy and come to terms with what I had just been through.

So at 3 pm on Friday, February 13, David brought me home to where I belong - with my family. At 5.30 I walked into a very messy and untidy house and knew that I was going to be around for just a little while longer.

I have been given a list of do's and don'ts for each week. This week it is a little light dusting, BUT next week I will class as the most exciting of all, because I am allowed to pot a plant!!

Now few people are less green-fingered than me, so this will be a whole new opportunity and as I am not meant to vacuum for another couple of weeks (but have done already), I will have to be very careful not to make a mess!

Well, it has been a bit of an epic this week but it is lovely to be back behind the computer again writing my diary. The only difference is that I now have this super new drainage system in my body. (Over a litre of fluid was drained from the sac around my heart, then an opening was made which now leads into my diaphragm, this in turn had a circle cut into it which will then drain fluid into my tummy and kidneys and then of course Mother Nature takes care of the rest.)

So, I am still here and not with my dad yet... am I lucky or am I lucky? Of course I would like to see my lovely old dad again, but maybe not just yet, eh?

Rhona x

March 1, 2004: *So, when is the best time to say goodbye?*

PLANT-potting week has arrived but have I done it? I'm afraid not, as I am suffering from sleepiness. Now that half term is over and I am at home by myself, I am finding it a struggle to stay awake. It has got so bad I was beginning to worry about it but have been assured by the professionals that it is only natural, as my body has been through a lot and is now trying to repair itself.

I want to return to my old life of lunching, decorating and, most of all, being a non-sleeping mum. Friends are coming to see me but I seem to tire after about an hour and then when they go I curl up on the sofa with a blanket and sleep for anything up to four hours. Honestly, what kind of life is that?

My breathing also hasn't improved much - I'm still very breathless after climbing the stairs. What amazes me is that, until the day I was discharged from hospital, I had continuous use of oxygen and was having four-hourly nebulisers. Then suddenly I was home with nothing. I have asked my Macmillan nurse to see if I can borrow a nebuliser, even for just a short period, to help my breathing during this time of convalescence. In the meantime, I will continue to dream of planting pots.

When David and the children came to visit me on the high-dependency wards, I was able to see the fear on their faces, as the realisation dawned that I didn't just have a cold, but a real-life terminal illness.

I didn't really think it would have much of a long-term effect on the children. How wrong I was.

Kristopher, in particular, is really struggling with confronting what is essentially any child's worst fear. Since coming home my lovely son has changed into the teenager I never imagined I would have. He is hurting, but with that, he is now very angry with me. He can see all of his friends having normal lives, with mums who do everyday normal things like staying awake.

He is beginning to realise he is not going to have a mum soon and with that, this time-bomb of a life will change for the worse.

It is very difficult to try not to scream back, when verbal abuse from my beloved son is becoming part our everyday lives.

How do I make a teenager whose heart is breaking understand that I too am hurting?

I don't want him to go through adult life with regrets about things he has said to me. It really isn't him talking but his anger that he is losing his mum, who he has always been able to count on for love, cuddles and kisses.

I know life will go on for my family when this is all over, as it did for me when my mum died, but, like many things in life, it is the waiting that is the worst part.

We all know that I am going to die, as to when, well of course we don't know, but I know I have most probably already lived the longest part of this "death sentence" - the

cancer was well and truly back in my body long before the official diagnosis. So that leaves us with the shorter part now but exact days and times aren't an option in the demise of a patient with cancer.

I'm not sure which is the best way to lose a parent. I have had it both ways a long illness with my mum when I was just 13 and a quick, unexpected death with my dad when I was 38.

When mum died, my life actually moved on quickly afterwards. I think it helped in that much of the

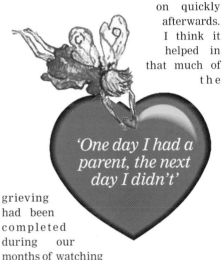

'One day I had a parent, the next day I didn't'

grieving had been completed during our months of watching her suffer. That, and the fact that she had turned into someone who wasn't my real mum. In many ways it was all a relief when it was over. As funerals then took place the day following a death in Ireland, the whole bereavement was over quite quickly.

With my dad, however, who was my much-loved friend for many years longer, we didn't have any notice of his heart attack - one day I had a parent and the next day I didn't.

After that, life changed. I would set myself goals to try to get myself that little bit further through each day before I cried - I couldn't believe the day when I reached lunchtime without tears.

So when is the best time to say goodbye?...I guess we will never know.

During the time I have been typing this, David and I have had numerous phone calls from an insurance company. Francesca is going on a skiing holiday with her school at Easter, so insurance being arranged between the school and us. However, as usual, the word "cancer" has thrown all those dealing with it into a flap!

I have had several callers, who seem to me to be 13- year-old boys, phone me and ask me to explain my medical condition. When I go through the cancers, they then ask me how they should categorise this.

Another asked me if I considered this to be life-threatening and then another asked me if I felt the need to see a doctor!! As this is my daughter's insurance and not my own, I would have always assumed that my health was of little or no relevance. Apparently it is in case something happens to me during her week away and she would not have the cover to enable her to come home.

We would never expect her school to have to deal with a situation like this anyway, as David would always fly to Switzerland to collect her and bring her back. Once again, it does bring it all home to us.

Insurance, on the whole, will be a nightmare for us from now on, so I don't think there will be any more long-haul trips for the Damants. At least we will now see the beauty our own country has offer.

I'm sure, having read this, you will think that I was born on a Wednesday as, after all, I seem to be full of woe right now. But guess what? I am a Sunday child so it is time to go and try to change myself into that bonny person. (I did say try...)

Rhona x

March 8, 2004: *At last I ve got a spring back in my step*

AFTER too many days in a black mood, things have started to look up for me...AT LAST!

I have managed to pick myself up and go for life again. No doubt another thunderbolt will hit me, maybe soon but hopefully later, but for now I'm wanting to be me again (OK, maybe a sleepier version!) I'm back to trying to enjoy what I can on a day-to-day basis.

So what happened...well lunch did . . . twice on consecutive days! One very close friend decided I needed an airing last Thursday, so we went out, had some lunch, then a little shopping in Lavenham. The following day another lovely friend had the same idea. As both days were freezing, I came back home with my cheeks slightly rosier than when I went out, getting my own colouring back at last!

On Saturday morning Francesca and a friend decided to have a practice run on the dry ski slope in Ipswich in preparation for their forthcoming school ski trip. As the weather was bitter and as it was also too early in the day for me I decided against going, but just as I was about to snuggle under the duvet for a second round of sleep of day I suddenly thought "What am I doing?" Here was my daughter's first skiing lesson and I wasn't going to see it, what on earth was I thinking about?

So within half an hour I was ready to go. It was a memorable morning with David capturing some of it on video. I must admit, although I watched her, it was from inside the bar with a huge glass of creamy chocolate, and not alongside the other parents who watched proudly by the slopes, but it is something else I have been able to watch my child achieve. Maybe "achieve" isn't quite the correct word to use, but I'm sure you know what I mean!

Sunday, however, was spent in bed recovering from the previous three days, but since it was almost three weeks since my surgery, I decided I would become "me" again and charge forward and attack life!

Monday brought the first of my spring cleaning days. I had received so many flowers during my unwell spell, but unfortunately by this stage the blooms were well past their best, so into the bin they went - along with all thought of what I had just been through! Of course I am not indestructible so I imagine there will still be bad days. Right now I am back on course to be around just that little bit longer for my family and friends.

'I'm on course to be around a little longer'

I had a phone call from a lady last week who reads my column. She, like me, has to watch some of her much-loved family suffer from this killer disease, but wanted to know if I had heard about the latest research and findings of the "Thalidomide" drug. I had briefly heard something on the radio, but in all honesty hadn't really taken any notice of it.

As I was a 1960s baby I had been told about the drug by my mum as she had been offered it for morning sickness, but had luckily turned it down.

This lady went on to tell me that some sorts of cancers have had a good response to the drug as it can reduce blood flow to the tumour. She wanted to tell me about it to see if I could be given the chance to try it.

Could I therefore please say thank you for thinking of offering me this opportunity to ask my consultant at the Marsden to listen to my pleas about it and let me have a go. If it doesn't work I have absolutely nothing to lose, but maybe a longer life to gain, to allow me some more time watching my children grow up.

Since that phone call, I have spent many hours on the internet finding out and printing off information, so when I go to hospital on March 11 I will be able to meet my doctor prepared with questions for when he tries to say the "no" word to me.

I think he often dreads moments like this, as when I hear research findings he knows that I will always be the one asking if I can go on that particular trial. I always seem to come away with a negative response - one day I'm sure he will find that have I the right type of cancer to have a go.

Today has been a lovely spring day and when I was in the garden with our dog I found my first little crocus. Spring is by far my favourite time of the year.

Many times recently I didn't think that I would see this season again, but here I am about to enter the time when David and I don't see to eye - you see I like to pick the daffodils in our garden, but he doesn't.

I can't really see the point in allowing their beauty to go unnoticed in the flower beds, so in my opinion, we should have vases of them all over the house. I think just to show I don't have any hard feelings about his disagreement with me, I will pick him the biggest bunch ever and put them by side of the bed for our wedding anniversary which is now just a few weeks away! (Another milestone.)

Anyway, before I finish this week, I wonder if you heard the story about an Irish woman and the friend who brought her a little bottle of champagne to celebrate her recent discharge from hospital?

Well, if you haven't, it finishes like this.

29

Between them they spent about 15 minutes trying to pop the cork, with the Irish one saying that she could hear the hissing of the cork being released.

It was only after several failed attempts they discovered that the cork was plastic, it just pulled and underneath was a screw cap which had to be opened by the Irish woman's son in front of two giggly but embarrassed close friends!

(No prizes for guessing who this story could be about!)

Rhona x

March 15, 2004: *Surviving the Titanic, and a box of champagne truffles*

WELL, I think that I am very much back on track to being me again (apart from a slight version of sleepy sickness). I now go back to bed for just two hours every morning after the children go to school and I'm up by 11am instead of mid-afternoon. Only four weeks after major surgery, things are looking up.

I am a strong believer in breakfast - even when I was sleeping into the afternoon, I would still have my cereal and orange when I got up - so I surprised myself last week when I ate a full box of champagne truffles instead, followed by a fizzy drink.

I would never allow my children to feast themselves on such a fancy diet. I think my brain is telling me to do the naughty things I want before it's too late! Lily, our Westie, decided to follow suit and next day ate a full box of Belgian liqueur chocolates, foils, box and all, which meant a night at the vet's having an injection to clear her tummy. It was a very expensive box of chocolates, but thankfully not my champagne truffles!

Francesca's school staged a wonderful version of *Titanic* last week. Stoke by Nayland Middle School has been fantastic to us. Their empathy, concern and kindness towards all of us is incredible, and in all honesty I dread the day in July when Francesca has to leave.

The day before we took our seats to watch more than 100 children perform, one of Francesca's teachers phoned to ask if I would like a comfy chair, which I accepted straight away, but then she said she had a sensitive issue to discuss with me.

As people arrived, they received a ticket telling them if they were first, second or third class passengers and at the end, they found out whether they died or not. Of course when I received mine the following night I found myself to be a third class passenger, so I died...but just as I was about to accept my fate, Kristopher insisted that we should swap, so David died and my son and I swam!

I'm sure most mums have experienced the nesting instinct just before their baby is born. I have always believed in instinct and lived my life accordingly. Now I find myself, just as I did years ago before K & F were born, going berserk trying to get things in order. I have sorted out my wardrobe, cupboards and all my personal things.

I know it will help David when the time comes, but I hope that, just this once, my instinct is wrong and I have just got the spring cleaning urge and am not about to pop off very soon.

I received a lovely letter the other day from a lady who I imagine to be quite young and is suffering from you-know-what. She, like me, is needle-phobic and is also having problems with her veins. We seem to share many of the same fears and thoughts.

She, however, is currently experiencing life without hair, and reading that made all my memories of those days come rushing back. For a female, I honestly believe that losing your hair has to be one of the worst things about having cancer. Treatment often results in the worst sickness that you will ever know, but the memories leave you quite quickly (as with giving birth - all the pain and discomfort is soon a distant memory). With chemo, there will be some bad days followed by just as many good, if not more before the next cycle.

A woman's hair, however, is the main feature of her face. If eyebrows and lashes also go, as mine did, then the whole feminine aspect is lost. I chose not to wear a wig and had my head shaved as soon as my hair started falling out.

It was David who asked me to do this, as it was coming out in clumps when I combed it, or else it would be on my pillow each morning which resulted in frequent tears.

My then neighbour, Margaret, took me to the hairdressers late one evening when everyone had gone and talked me through watching my thick, blonde hair falling to the floor. As it happened, David's decision was the right one, as when it's gone it's gone!

Friends came hat shopping with me, so very soon I had a colourful collection for all occasions. Given that most women who live their lives under hats are nearly always doing so for the same reason, it is surprising how many people out there are still cruel or make stupid remarks. I can remember many glares, stares and nods in my direction, especially in restaurants.

Before I had cancer, I never looked because, from my own background, I knew the reason behind the hats and scarves. Unfortunately there will always be someone out there who thinks a sideways glance will go unnoticed. For the cancer sufferer, I'm afraid it doesn't.

Just one last word to that lovely brave lady - your hair will come back in time, but be aware it will be different from your last hair. Mine came back very fine but with a definite curl to it. Although I tried the cold cap (a hair-preserving process that some hospitals use. I will ask the Marsden this week and write more about it all next time as the technology has progressed quite a lot since then and I want to get the facts completely right) it didn't really work for me and my hair started to fall out two weeks after my first cycle of chemo.

I started using it again on my fifth cycle, however, and by the time I finished my sixth and last one I had quite a covering of hair all over my head. Four weeks after that I had my first trim! I kept with my very short haircut for quite some time as it didn't make my face look so drawn but once I started to gain weight I decided I wanted to look like the old me again.

My heart goes out to those who are experiencing this right now. I know exactly how you feel, but, as many friends used to say to me, at least I never had a bad hair day!

Always remember that you are still you - hair or not (as everyone used to remind me on a daily basis).

Although it is easy to say and often difficult to carry out, ignore the funny looks and try to concentrate on all the positive things that life has to offer.

Rhona x

March 22, 2004: *An unpleasant week, all in all*

WHAT a week! Two hospital appointments in London, a hungover dog, some travel trials, and of course shopping, lunch and lots of sleep!

People think when you become terminally ill with cancer life will stop there and then, but how much more excitement could there possibly be? Lily is now well after her

31

afternoon on liqueur chocolates, but for two days she slept, obviously sleeping off her hangover - though I don't think it will have taught her a lesson!

One of the perks of being so ill is having an ambulance car to get to the Marsden every three weeks, operated by The East Anglian Ambulance Service. The drivers are so wonderful, I cannot praise them highly enough.

As the Royal Brompton Hospital is about a minute away from the Marsden, I was surprised to hear that transport for my after-surgery appointment would be provided by another company. When I asked why, I was told that it was a way of saving money and that budgets had to be adhered to. Who am I, or anyone else for that matter, to argue against this? We all know that unfortunately everything in the medical world depends on budgets.

The transport was arranged through my doctor's surgery and I was told that my car would pick me up on Wednesday at 11am. As this car was coming from London to collect me, then take me to the Brompton, wait for me, bring me back home again and then drive another three hours back to London, it meant a total of around 12 hours driving - instead of about seven hours for a local driver.

How can it be cheaper for a London company to do this rather than my own drivers?

'He said I should try to forget I was ill'

Yet it is. Anyway, on the morning in question I went into the shower at 9.45am, came out at 10am and guess what...the driver had been and gone! I know he can't have rung my doorbell, as Lily always lets us know if someone is at the door and she hadn't moved from the kitchen. I found a scrap of paper on the floor telling me he had been.

Both the doctor's surgery and I immediately rang the transport company, but were told that the driver wouldn't be returning. Besides, how was it that I had been in the shower when surely I knew their policy of being ready for at least an hour before my transport was due? (Mmm.. no!).

I asked the transport manager to phone me back, which he eventually did do. He constantly referred to me as "darlin'" and went on to tell me that they had cancelled my appointment!

Here I am trying to live a stress-free life and stay calm no matter what. So was I calm? Absolutely not! Eventually David drove me to London for my follow-up.

The consultant was pleased with my progress, handed me back to the care of the Marsden and told me to go home, have a beer and forget that this had ever happened! He went on to say that I should now lead a proper life and try to forget that I was ill. Well of course that is easy, isn't it?

Thursday was Marsden day and it was a relief to have my own friendly driver back again. They found a vein first time and as I had kept the "wimp cream" on for over an hour before the cannula was inserted, I actually did not feel it. After five years, I have finally sussed that the anaesthetic cream only works properly after an hour.

I had a list of questions for my consultant but was told he had left to focus on research. This was quickly followed by the news that the consultant in charge of my over all care, who deals purely with breast cancer secondaries, had lost his own wife, aged 40, from breast cancer the weekend before.

How devastating for this doctor, but also for women like me, because from a selfish point of view, where does that leave us? If a woman cannot be saved from this disease when her husband is the top consultant at the main cancer hospital, what hope is there for the rest of us?

I have now been handed over to yet another doctor - the sixth in nine months. As I wasn't quite prepared for this, I felt awkward asking her my many questions. I did ask about the Thalidomide drug trial, however and she said she had used this before for treatment but never for breast cancer.

I had all my facts ready and she did say she would try to find out further details and get back to me - but I won't be waiting for that phone to ring.

In the meantime, I was advised to take life easy, remember how ill I am and to try to be as stress-free as possible, whereas the day before I was being told by the Brompton I had to forget I was ill. From where I am sitting that seems very much like two conflicting pieces of advice. Do I wrap myself in cotton wool and wallow in self-pity or do I risk all infections and enjoy what is left of my life? No prizes for guessing which option I've decided to go for!

Anger and bitterness haven't ever really been factors over the past five years. I haven't dwelled on how it is that I can have been allowed to get in this state given my family history of breast cancer deaths.

One of the nicest things that happened all week was a lovely surprise waiting for me on my return home after my drip. It was a beautiful bunch of daffodils from a couple who, although they live quite close, I have never actually met. Their kindness brought some spring sunshine to what was otherwise quite an unpleasant week.

I wrote last week about the chemotherapy cold cap or scalp-cooling as it is now known. When I was given this treatment I had my head wrapped in bandages with bags of ice placed on top. The treatment has proved very successful with certain types of drugs (doxorubicin, epirubcin and taxotere). The aim is to cool the scalp so the coldness narrows the blood vessels and prevents the drug passing into the cells at the hair root and damaging them. The cap, which resembles those worn by jockeys, is obviously very cold, quite heavy and can feel uncomfortable.

First the hair is dampened with a wet bandage placed around the head and cotton pads around the ears to protect them from the cold. The cap is then placed on the head for 15 minutes before the start of chemotherapy and will stay on for 45 minutes after the drug has been given.

Often, replacement caps are used depending on the length of treatment. I never found them to be very glamorous, but if it works…well what the heck?

Rhona x

March 29, 2004: *Great start, bad finish*

LAST week started off great but became one that I didn't like at all. On Wednesday, Tony and Natalie from Anglia Television arrived to finish off filming for a documentary.

As we didn't get much from the Marsden hospital earlier in the year, my doctor very kindly agreed to talk about my situation. I was having quite a few problems with headaches anyway, so much of the filming was on what would have been a routine appointment. He did, however, finish with talking about cancer in general.

I have a very understanding doctor, who

in my 13 years of being his patient has shown compassion. As he knows me much better than the many doctors at the hospital I think it was only right it was he who had the final word on me.

It is quite sad all of this has now come to an end, as "Tone and Nat" have become such good friends. I obviously won't see them as much, but we do intend to "do lunch" from time to time.

Everyone has a Christmas card list for new friends and acquaintances, but I have a "funeral list". So, sorry you two, but I've just added your names to it!

Thursday was a very exciting day. Katy Edwards came over early to discuss a feature I wanted to do as a thank you to all the lovely people who write to me, helping to keep my spirits up. Later, Dominic Castle (EADT deputy editor) and Julian Ford (features editor) joined us, so the four of us went to Lavenham for lunch.

I have always said how it is impossible to find a book about an everyday mum having to cope with terminal cancer, a book which has the answers to frequently asked questions, the real insight of playing a waiting game and, of course, the many ups and downs of living with the "Big C".

This is what my diary is all about.

Now, with the help of the EADT, my dreams of seeing this book in print could very soon come true. It is early days, but we have discussed many aspects of the project. I have decided all proceeds would go to the genetic screening department of the Royal Marsden and Suffolk Breakthrough, in the hope that, when the time comes, things will have moved on so much that my children will have a healthier future.

That night was the start of my bleak week. I have read that often people who have brain tumours lose confidence and become panicky and muddled. I have never thought too much about this as it just wouldn't happen to me.

Or would it? Well, unfortunately it did, without me at first realising it.

I went to bed on Thursday night much earlier than normal because I felt very tired and actually very sore in various parts of my body. I woke up Friday feeling terrible, but in all honesty have experienced this feeling so many times before I tried to dismiss it.

I had to go shopping at the local supermarket and left the house as "me" but reached the car park, picked up a trolley and froze. Suddenly I couldn't see anything, my ears were ringing, I thought I was going to be sick, I started shaking, felt faint and knew I had lost all of colour in my face. Fortunately there were only a few essential items on my list so I quickly picked them up (except that they weren't the ones actually on my list), paid for them and rushed to the car. I sat in the car park for quite some time and then it hit me.

This was the first time in the last nine months that I had gone anywhere so busy by myself. Over the past months the tumours in my brain have decided upon themselves to put green wellies on and trample all over my self confidence. Of course, as it happened without me knowing that it was going to happen, it was all very scary. No doubt in the future I will be wary of being by myself in crowded environments. The "me" I have known for the last 43 years is now a distant memory.

For the next four days I remained in bed with an all-singing, all-dancing bout of flu, my temperature was so high that when I was asleep I kept dreaming Tony Blair was sending me birthday cards!

Now, if you are a man reading this, maybe you would like to skip the next few paragraphs. Up until last June I had been taking the "wonder drug" Tamoxifen. My breast cancer was categorised and confirmed as oestrogen receptor positive, which simply meant I had too much of that hormone in

34

in my body. So to hopefully stop it from happening again I was given this drug as it is an "anti oestrogen", meaning any future breast tumours could not feed from this.

There were many side-effects but apart from one I managed to get over them quite quickly. But it is always the horrible one that seems to remain and, in my case, it was an early menopause.

How wonderful! I have suffered hot flushes, night sweats, and mood swings (oh, and aren't they lovely!) After four years on this drug I was relieved when at last I was taken off it last year.

OK, my cancer had returned but at least no more red faces in restaurants and windows wide open in the middle of winter. My menopause was over!

But guess what? NOW I am going through the REAL menopause. Does anyone know where I can buy some laughing tablets? GENTLEMEN - you can come back now.

Just one last moan (afraid so!) I have a disabled parking badge, which has been a bit of an eye-opener. Before I had the authority to park in one of those spaces I would never have considered using one for my convenience. On recent occasions, I have found it irritating to find that nearly always the allocated spaces have been used, often by people without badges. Can I just say to those people who do this: please do not be jealous of people like me who do need to be close to supermarkets, etc.

Life has dealt us an unfair hand with our health and by having this privilege it can make our lives just a little easier. I would gladly give up my disabled authorisation if I could only have some of my good health back.

Well, I'm off to buy a card for my newfound friend, the prime minister. Maybe I should put him on my list.....

Rhona x

April 5, 2004: *It s OK to be a fishwife*

I WOULD like to thank Katy Edwards for organising a great health column last week. I told her I would say thank you every week in my diary to everyone for all their cards and letters. But I wanted to do more, to tell everyone how much all of this means to me.

So I lent my precious box to Katy and gave her the very difficult job of putting it all together. Obviously, as space was limited it would have been an impossible task for all of them to be printed. There was absolutely no way that I could ever choose as they all mean so much to me.

Since lending my treasures to the EADT, I have received two further letters, one which brought me much laughter and sunshine to what was a rather dull day. This was from a nun, who wrote: "You are allowed to feel resentful, to be angry, to think and feel what you like, and if it helps, have a Billingsgate fishwife row with the good Lord over the situation."

I have quoted this to most of my friends and I want them to share in my laughter and I want to share it with you, too.

I have my own beliefs on religion and think it should be a private matter left to the individual. As a child, I was always sent to Sunday school wearing my best dress, gloves, and hat. As I became older my church attendance became confined to life's bigger events like weddings, christenings and midnight mass on Christmas Eve.

My poor attendance, of course, didn't change my beliefs, except for a while after my mum died. My dad, however, went in the other direction and became a very religious person. Cancer was such a taboo word in the early 1970s. I felt ashamed and embarrassed that I had lost my mum to this thing. For years I found it easier to tell everyone that my parents had divorced and my mum had gone to live in France. A far-fetched story for a normal little Irish girl, I know. As a result, I couldn't speak about my feelings for God to anyone. The separation of parents shouldn't make you dislike God the way I did.

For a very long time I lived in a muddle over all of this, and to a degree probably still do a little today. That is why this great letter - almost 30 years since my mum's death and almost five years since the start of my own cancer - has brought me such release. At least I now feel it is OK to question all of this and become that "fish-wife".

My thoughts have changed since the word "terminal" was first mentioned. I now have confidence that my parents are waiting for me and I will be able to look after my family after my death. I have accepted the fact that I will go when the time is right and no amount of hedging my bets can change that. What I am really now doing is what my dad did when he lost his soulmate, and I think, in turn, my children are now doing what I did.

The other letter was so much sadder but a great comfort to me nonetheless because it told me I was achieving what I set out to do in writing my diary - to be an inspiration to others when times are bad.

This was a letter from a man who was fulfilling his late wife's wish of wanting to write to me, as she too had tumours in her brain and lungs.

Unfortunately, her condition worsened very quickly and she lost her fight in February, but even though this man is still in the very early stages of his grieving process he took the time to write to me. I am not going to repeat all those clichés that peo-ple tend to say after the death of a much-loved person, except to say that I will think of you often and hope that, in time, life will start to look up for you again just in the same way that I hope it will for my family when they have to go through what you are now.

I have many friends dotted around the world from my long-haul flying days. Over the years, contact with many of them has turned to the yearly Christmas card and maybe the odd telephone call. Towards the end of last week, I had a surprise call from Anna, a Norwegian friend who I last saw in 1994 when we paid her a visit.

She phoned to tell me that she had just divorced her third husband! As the conversation went on, I mentioned that my cancer had returned and when I told her where, a huge silence descended. I knew what she was thinking. Death, and soon!

Two days later she phoned to say that she was arriving that weekend. (Silly girl, how dare she think I was about to go in the next week!) When she arrived I knew from the relief on her face when she saw me that she realised I wasn't quite at death's door.

We had a great three days together; but must admit I will now pay for my frivolous partying (staying up to 1am talking). I will miss her as she came over as a guest but insisted on doing everything, even bringing me my early morning cuppa.

Just as it was with Diane, who I said goodbye to in Sydney in the New Year, promises are always made to meet up soon - but it is only a ploy to stop the tears. Diane is too far away, and although Anna is now single again she is a career person. I must be honest with myself and admit that these were actually the final goodbyes.

Kristopher has recently had some more counselling from the St Nicholas Hospice in Bury St Edmunds. Initially it made some difference to his angry attitude, but it seems his bitterness is returning. Francesca is away skiing for the first week of the school holidays, so I hope that my boy and I will be able to have many mother-and-son chats.

My flu has gone and the sun has come out. Before I dropped Anna at the train station we sat outside a pub having lunch. The saying "It's good to be alive" came to mind, and it was the first time I had stopped to think about its true meaning.

So, it's back to the good old Royal Marsden this week for my bone-drip. Most people will be tucking into hot cross buns on Friday, but I will have a bruised arm and tiredness. It is unlikely chemo will be mentioned but I wouldn't be surprised if I have an MRI soon. During my last visit I told the consultant of recurring pins and needles and numbness in my right hand. Since then it has got worse and is now starting to affect my left hand. It also happens when I bend my head. They might put it down to recent radiotherapy damage (they usually do). I hope not, though, because it is concerning me, and I would like it to be further investigated before I lose all the power in my hands permanently.

Well, this brings me to wishing you all a great Easter and to urge you to eat as many chocolate eggs as you can. I certainly will. Why worry about diets when enjoying life is so much more fun!

Rhona x

April 12, 2004: *I'm starting to hate this new, daft me*

I hope the Easter bunny paid everyone a visit with bags of eggs, and that diets were once again forgotten for another week!

I expect most people are now saying "spring has sprung" but my brain is becoming quite muddled. I am saying something like "sprung has springed!" I am now beginning to find, especially when I am tired, that the words which I want to say are all coming out wrong and most sentences will either take me a while to complete or are spoken in a language alien to the rest of this world, including myself.

I usually manage to laugh it off with friends but, in actual fact, it is annoying, irritating and frustrating to me, especially when I think of this daft person I am turning into, a person I am beginning to hate.

I have come to the conclusion, after too many times waking up during the night, that I am now getting tired of this cancer thing and have decided that, even if offered, I won't have any further poisonous treatment. My bone-drip is something I need to control the pain, and my body is now used to any side-effects, but anything new will bring with it all the things, like sickness, that I have experienced in the past. It is quality of life I want now and not quantity - and I don't think even David will

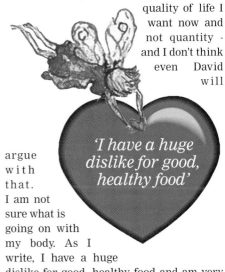

'I have a huge dislike for good, healthy food'

argue with that.

I am not sure what is going on with my body. As I write, I have a huge dislike for good, healthy food and am very happy with eating silly things. I hate 6pm as I know it is getting close to the time that I am going to have to eat a meal. David is doing all the cooking now, but I hate the fact that he comes home after a full day at work, cooks - and then I throw most of it away. It is really quite a relief when it is all over. I am still going out just as much for lunch, but I am finding that sandwiches or part of a jacket potato is as much as I can manage.

However, I can eat any amout of sweet things, whereas in the past that was my daughter and not me. Today I went to one of my favourite eating places (Corncraft in Monks Eleigh) and tucked into a huge fresh cream strawberry meringue which filled me up so much I didn't want any dinner, but to me that was much better than any meat and two veg.

Anyway, enough of Rhona's moans and groans!

I had a great day out last weekend at the Ideal Home Exhibition in London with a great friend. I surprised myself with the strength I seemed to have for the entire day (I did suffer, though, all day Sunday and ended up with a very bad breathing attack that evening).

I bought so many things for the house, including stunning duvet covers for K & F's beds. I rarely seem to buy anything for myself now. Again, it seems to be a nesting instinct, making sure the house will be perfect for my family when this DIY enthusiast has made her departure.

The day was one of giggles and silliness, but then I had the absolute worst compliment of my life. Apart from having a ring cleaned, a makeover and my hair straightened, I also had my shoes cleaned. The teenager doing it made a good job and then said that he wished he was 30 years older! The smile soon disappeared from my face when I realised that, in his wisdom, he thought I was approaching my half century!

Now, were it not for my great fear of needles, I think I would have gone straight away to find some botox injections!

I watch *Holby* each Tuesday night, not because of the fact that it always seems to have someone who has cancer on it (and nearly always dies!) but because I am in love with Owen. As I watched it last week a comment was made which had to be one of the best I have ever heard - "Regret is just a wasted emotion."

Isn't that just so true? How many silly things in life have we all wasted precious time worrying about? Of course we will all carry on doing just as we have always, but wouldn't it be so lovely if regret wasn't in our vocabulary?

As I write I am getting ready for my hospital visit. I have a friend going with me this time, which will give David a break, but will also be quite an eye-opener for her.

The medical day unit is mostly a ward for chemo, but other treatments are given, such as blood transfusions and bone-drips. It is quite a colourful room (a bit too orange for my liking, but at least not an old-fashioned, sickly, hospital green).

Most people would think it is a place for sad, depressed, self-denying people, but it is not! Instead it can often be quite loud with laughter, but never tears. The staff know all their patients with their likes and dislikes, and we are all scared of the lady who serves us with our tea and then the stale, tasteless sandwich at lunchtime.

We often see people we haven't seen before, but we never ask the reason why

'Regret is just a wasted emotion'

people don't appear again. There is also the great benefit of reading all the latest magazines without having to buy them. But most of all, we are all the same, regardless of age, hair (or lack of it), gender or beauty. Each of us having one thing in common, we are all trying desperately to keep fighting the battle to live.

During my last visit I met a lovely girl there with her dad. She was very beautiful, young, chatty and healthy-looking, so I was amazed to find it was her and not her dad who had cancer. I heard her chatting to a doctor who answered her questions on the secondaries in her brain which followed very quickly after her first diagnosis of breast cancer. The age of this girl? Just 18 years old.

Once again it is a reminder that the current programme of offering mammograms only after the age of 50 is wrong. The recent extension of allowing women over the age of 70 to have this yearly check is not going to alter the statistical fact that breast cancer is killing more and more younger women.

Adverts on the TV and in the newspapers urging people to donate generously to cancer research is not going to lower deaths unless the first move is made to make screening available to the under-50 age group too.

Even though I had a family history I wasn't automatically put forward for checks. If I had been on a reminder list my lump would have been detected very early on and I would now be living a life with a future. It would be nice to meet up with this girl again but no one will volunteer any information if she is not there.

Then, after a short period of time, she will be forgotten like so many before her, because those with memory problems resulting from brain tumours tend to forget things and often don't remember them again.

Well, I am off to meet my old friends "Tone and Nat" from Anglia Television to discuss further filming for the documentary. We all thought two weeks ago that was it, we had finished, but just as I was returning to normal (??) life again, Natalie phoned up. So I'm off to practice my Oscar-winning speech and work out a way to perfect my tears. Well, if Gwyneth Paltrow can do it, so can I.

Rhona x

April 19, 2004: *I m feeling so vulnerable*

IAM sorry to say I haven't liked this past week either and am beginning to wonder if I am ever going to have the energy to enjoy a full week again.

This is the first time I have found myself actually struggling with the words typing this diary. My concentration level seems to be quite low and trying to re-read what I have just written is taking an age. I always write a little letter to Katy (Edwards) before my column, which today has taken me about ten times longer to get to make sense, so I do hope this column will.

People often speak about miracles. I have been told on many occasions they do happen but, in all honesty, I have never really put a lot of thought into whether they do or not.

However, during last week a miracle did happen; unfortunately not for me, but for a special little girl. During our time in Australia, you may remember that I met a very lovely friend of mine, Diane. She and her partner have two gorgeous girls, Tayla, seven, and Olivia, just two. Both girls are very pale; Diane, like many Australians, has suffered from skin cancer in the past. With their sun being as strong as it is, the girls

39

are always either covered up or have the highest sun factor cream spread all over their little bodies, so it never crossed our minds that one of them could be sick.

It was a month after our return that Diane phoned with the news that Tayla was quite ill, TB being the likely diagnosis. The news then came that this tiny blonde beauty had lymphoma and things did not look good. She went on to spend five full weeks on a children's cancer ward with continuous drips feeding into her little veins. Diane was at her side at all times.

At the end of this treatment Tayla had a scan. The results showed Tayla had no sign of this cancer in her body. The oncologists said they had never seen a child leave that cancer ward with only two band-aids, having had extensive cancer only a few weeks before. Tayla was then booked in a few days later to have her lungs re-inflated, as one had totally collapsed and the other partially. When she went in and was scanned, her lungs were perfect.

This story is the stuff of dreams but in this case it has been a definite miracle - they do happen after all. When I spoke to Tayla last week she told me that she was good and that her lungs were "better forever" now.

If a miracle is to happen, it is right it should happen to a child, as no child should be robbed of a life. Diane has said she wishes I could have this sort of miracle. I do too, but I know I will have to be happy just knowing it happened to Tayla.

It was funny that I wrote last week, praising my hospital. The following day, when I went up for my bone-drip visit, was a disaster. There was a new nurse, who seemed very confident. I know my own veins and those that can still give blood for testing. She decided that others that haven't worked for months should be used.

As I started to feel very nervous with her, I explained there were certain nurses who canulate me each time and that I have built up all my confidence in them over a long period of time. I was, and still am, feeling very vulnerable as I know my cancer is progressing.

Although I have kept the tearful moments for David and myself so far, I could feel myself falling apart as she told me that I didn't have the right to choose and therefore it would be her whether I liked it or not. By this time I was feeling so sick, knowing there would be problems with the needle. I spoke to one of the more senior nurses who is one of my "calmers down". She told me not to worry, as someone else would do it. I wasn't quite ready, however, for what was to come.

In front of everyone, I was told by this so-called caring nurse that I irritated her more than she has ever been irritated before. Her shouting, my embarrassment and my unwell state seemed to go on forever, with her telling me I would have to wait an hour before I would be seen by another nurse. I said that was fine, but didn't expect to have to wait for two.

I had arrived on the medical day unit at 9am and was finally ready for my drip at 1.30pm. My alarm went off that morning at 5am, my drip finally finished at 5.30pm and I arrived back home close to 8.30pm. I expect to have long days at the hospital as it is my choice to travel to London but I don't think I deserve this sort of treatment.

I did also see a doctor that day, who organised a CT scan for me, but as there a waiting list, this won't be until May 18. She has said to bring David along for moral support when I get the results, but think I know what they will be, even before I have the scan. My cough is getting worse, there is more loss of power in my hands (radiotherapy damage), extreme tiredness, lack of appetite, pain in various parts of my body, headaches and nausea, so it doesn't take a lot of working out.

Louise (my best friend) and her family came down from Manchester for the Easter break. This is a long-standing tradition, with us going out on the Sunday to Lavenham to buy silly things for the four children and then adding those to the eggs for an Easter hunt. This is followed by a turkey roast dinner and pudding at about 11pm.

This year, tradition broke. I spent all Sunday in bed ill. We didn't get to buy the silly things, David and Jim hid all of the eggs and the children spotted them, just by walking down the garden. David had forgotten to take the turkey out to defrost, so dinner was thrown together from whatever could be found in the only shop that was open close by. Oh, and pudding was forgotten until the next night.

Maybe it is just as well that the tradition was broken this year, as next year I don't think there will be a choice.

Well, the noisy one is home from skiing, thankfully without any broken bones and looking very tanned (at least I think that is what it is!). Kristopher and I had a lovely week together. The two of us just enjoyed being with each other and I know it did both of us good, just having each other's company. I also don't seem to be bankrupt, which I suppose means that I was just happy to be with my son and him with his mum.

Kristopher, since starting upper school last September, has met up with various children he hasn't seen for many years, as they all went to different primary or middle schools. It has been lovely to see those friendships rekindled and that all the children are now old enough to understand what is happening with me, so I know when they come around I don't have to make excuses for how I look or feel.

There is one particular girl we have known since she was two - she was Kristopher's first girlfriend, when they were both three. Now, many years on, she has stepped back into our lives, so I would just like to thank Laura (a beautiful redhead) for being there for Kris, for her lovely specially chosen card for me, for her gentleness in talking to me when I haven't felt well and for being one of my greatest fans.

Francesca is having a joint 13th birthday party this weekend with her best friend Rosie, so all I can say is I hope I will have the strength to write my diary next week. If not, you will know I will probably have been sent to a faraway land - as my punishment for being too "uncool" on the dance floor.

When it is my turn on the karaoke, I will of course have to sing my version of *I will Survive*. After all, it is a mum's right to make their children hide their heads in shame, isn't it?

Rhona x

April 26, 2004: *Caron s death opened the floodgates*

I NORMALLY try to write my diary during a Tuesday, but this week it is Wednesday night and quite late.

During those 24 hours little things have changed, so this is now a completely different version to what it would have been on Tuesday.

Anyway, first things first...the party!! As you can see I am not off playing Robinson Crusoe on some paradise island, which means only one thing, I did not manage to sufficiently embarrass my children at Francesca and Rosie's 13th birthday party.

In fact, I didn't really get much of a chance to get on the floor at all or sing to the karaoke as the DJ we hired for the evening was an absolute disaster! He played only music he liked (awful), but worst of all, when it came to singing, he took his own microphone, wouldn't let anyone else have a go and squealed like a cat in pain for the rest of the night! Due to this man's silliness at the end, I didn't get to bed until 1.45am, which sent me on a downward spiral for the next few days.

I can't quite tell you exactly when it was that the floodgates opened and the tears came and lasted for far too long. As silly as it may sound, I think it was shortly after Caron Keating died. Of course, I never knew her, but like me, she was a Northern Irish girl and Gloria Hunniford was a household name as I was growing up - I can even remember her coming to my primary school.

After Caron died, I became obsessed with reading every possible paper trying to find out more; how she died and where her cancer had spread. After all, she died with the same disease that I am still trying very hard to fight.

My mind, after almost five years, became full of nothing but cancer and death. In the past couple of weeks, the pain has heightened in more parts of my body and the fatigue is so strong that when I am actually awake, I become quite excited about going back to sleep.

Sunday, Monday and Tuesday have honestly been the worst days that I have ever, ever had in my life. The tears wouldn't stop.

Francesca kept pleading with me to stop crying, telling me how much she hated it

'My mind became full of nothing but cancer and death'

and how it made her cry. I found myself telling Kristopher to remember that when I died I would be with his beloved "Gramps" and to look for the brightest star at night, when he was upset, because that would be me looking after him. Naturally this made him cry, and that made me worse.

It didn't matter what David said, he just could not console me. Mad and stupid thoughts would not leave my mind.

Three days is a long time to carry on in such a mad way. Thankfully on Tuesday, one of my closest friends phoned unexpectedly and when she heard the state I was in, came over half an hour later.

Our afternoon started off in tears, but ended up with smiles, thanks to her.

As I said earlier, it is now Wednesday night and I have reached a turning point. I have decided to return to Colchester hospital for the rest of my treatment, as I know my days at the Marsden have come to an end.

It was the right thing to do in the earlier days, being a patient at the top cancer hospital, pioneering all the latest treatments. I was cured, and went on to have a good, positive and healthy two years. I know that a cure will never be found for me now; the only thing left is symptom control.

Also the travelling to London is now sending me to bed for anything up to three days after my drip and I can no longer cope with the 5am starts. A journey of just 20 minutes up the road to a hospital seems a better option.

I have also spoken to my doctor and asked him for more help with the pain. He has sent off a plea to the Marsden in the hope that they will prescribe something. I have been given a painkiller that sends me to the moon when I take it and morphine has also been mentioned but I am not ready yet to lose my senses or hit the "hard stuff" as when that happens, there will be no going back.

Today, my friend who arrived when I was in a complete mess took me out to Bury for lunch and at last, I sort of became me again.

Now, had this been last night, I would still be in that hysterical state and that would have been where my diary would have ended.

Today things have changed thanks to three things, First, my friend being there for me at the right time, then a box of beautiful flowers being delivered to me by an EADT reader (can I please say a huge thank you to Christine for your most gorgeous and generous thoughts and gift - I love flowers so much, but I just can't believe you took the time to do this for me...you must be a very special lady).

The third was a phone call from a gentleman who had sent me a beautiful, tiny Bible his mum had given him. I knew it meant a lot to him and when I received it I felt so very emotional that someone could do something like this for me.

This Bible has been given a new home beside my bed, and in the future will be handed on to my children. His phone call helped give me some of my fight back and during our conversation I became aware that my mum and dad are looking after me, and have been during the past five years. This gentleman believes that I have the sheer determination to go on and pot my plants for many years. I'm not so sure, but I hope he is right and I am VERY wrong.

I am sure that my feeling better again is because I know so many people care for me, and I owe it to them and my family to get back into that boxing ring and fight once again.

I always have a little word up above every night before I go to sleep, and usually I ask for guidance. After today, however, I think I will say from now on: "Hey, no more tears please, help turn me back to the old Rhona days."

I did buy all of the papers again to read all about Caron Keating's funeral, even though most of them said the same, but I had to keep reading just in case I found any answers.

Of course I didn't but I sat for ages just looking at all the pictures thinking of how beautiful and serene it all seemed to be. More than anything, when my time comes this is how I would like my final farewell; a day of memories and laughter.

Well, that has brought me to my goodbyes for this week, so I'm just going off to have a word about waterproof mascara. That will give my dad something to think about won't it?

Rhona x

May 3, 2004: *I know the cancer is running riot now*

I feel as if the Marsden are washing their hands of me. I've spent a whole week on the phone to them trying to get someone to return my calls to speak about symptom control and arranging my CT scan.

I had a scan booked for my son's birthday (Monday, April 26) - I asked them not to, but when did they book it for? Monday - so I had to try to change it.

The pain started over a week ago. I phoned my GP; he said he would phone them and ask for an urgent CT scan for me and try to get pain relief. He sent a fax through but no one got back to me. I'm not sleeping at night with the pain in my neck, my ribs, my legs. It's been absolutely horrendous.

I then spoke to my Macmillan nurse and she phoned up (the Marsden) continuously and didn't get anywhere. She tried all day on Monday. They promised to get back to me, but didn't. Tuesday I phoned again. My

GP sent another fax through. We heard nothing. We had gone eight days without hearing anything, so on Tuesday at 4pm I phoned yet again and said I needed to speak to someone - I didn't care who - and that this was getting ridiculous.

An Irish doctor (not my usual doctor) phoned me back. She was really great. She said she'd try to book me in for a CT scan for next Tuesday or Wednesday and told me I could up my pain medication.

Then I got someone on Wednesday who said they'd booked me in the following day at 9am. I was due to go away with my family and there was no transport arranged (to get to the Marsden) or anything. Also they'd overbooked me, which I knew would mean I would have been in at 9am and would have had to wait most of the day. So I told them I couldn't do it. They turned around and said 'OK, it's your life, if it was so urgent you would go'. I wish I'd been quicker and thought to say that of course it was urgent - that was why I had been trying for 10 days to arrange the CT scan.

Now they've told me they can't get me in until May 18. I couldn't believe this doctor didn't answer my calls. It's been a nightmare. I'm up for another bone-drip next Thursday. I was hoping I would get the results of my CT scan that day then they could get me onto some sort of pain relief and we could talk about what treatment I could have from then on.

I'm no further forward. My GP has said it's not advisable to try to transfer (my care) to Colchester until I get this sorted.

My cancer is so obviously progressing. I know it's now running riot in me. I'm sure of it. I know my own body. I have this continuous tiredness. I get up to get the children to school, I don't even stay up with them to have their breakfast. The moment I hear them close the door I'm asleep again.

I can't climb the stairs without getting breathless. I'm so tired. I can't begin to explain the tiredness. I don't want to do anything. To walk to the end of the garden is an absolute miracle. I got the vacuum cleaner out four days ago but it's still in the middle of the floor. I haven't been able to do anything. There's no power in my hands. Until I get the scan results they can't tell me what's happening and whether I can get on a treatment.

I feel as if they are literally now just letting me go. My feelings are that the drug I want is probably too expensive. I know I said I didn't want any more chemo but lately I've been feeling that I want to go back on the chemo drug Capecitabine I had last year because I had such a good response from that. I can't go out at the moment. With Capecitabine I went from being so ill and close to dying to leading a normal life again and the tumours shrunk.

I've been told I can't have that again but I've contacted an oncologist in the U.S. who's said you can have it a second time, it should work, but a third time might not work. I've had no cancer treatment at all for six months except a bone-drip, which is just a calcium treatment. The drugs can't be in my body any longer so they should allow me to have it again. They say they can't do anything until I've had a CT scan. My thoughts are that it is probably money. The anti-sickness medication alone is about £10 a tablet.

As for the doctor who promised me two months ago that she would be there for me, she can't even answer my phone calls. It's just so rude. It's completely worn me out, the feeling that they're just not bothering. It's absolutely horrendous.

May 18 is still a long way away, I need something to stop this pain. I can't even turn over in bed at night. When I try to get out of bed I'm like an old woman. I'm shuffling about because I can't walk properly with the pain. The Marsden is supposed to

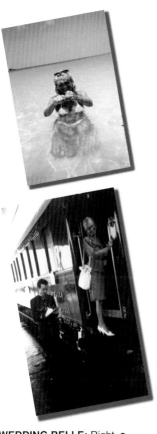

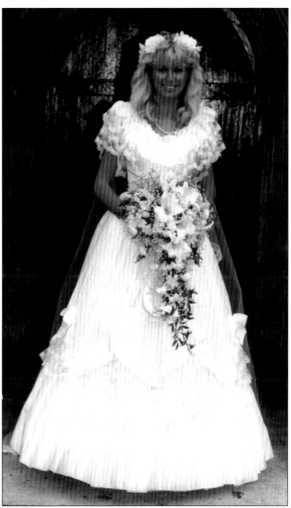

WEDDING BELLE: Right, a radiant Rhona at her wedding at Hintlesham Church in 1988. Above, showing off her engagement ring in Antigua and she's off on honeymoon on the Orient Express

STYLE AND FUN: Left, Rhona and David at David's sister's wedding at Hintlesham Church in 1987. Right, Rhona gets the giggles on the morning of her own wedding with bridesmaid Louise

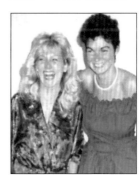

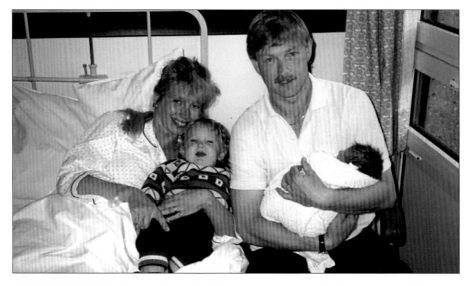

FAMILY COMPLETE: Rhona with David, Kristopher and new arrival Francesca in 1991

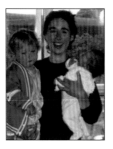

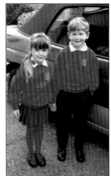

LITTLE ANGELS:
The bundles of joy
with midwife Gina
and, right, it's off to
Long Melford
Primary School

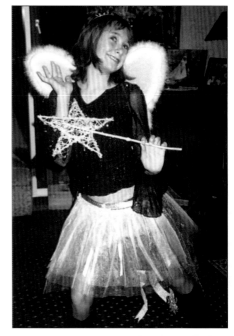

**A VERY GOOD
COMPANION:**
Lily the Westie,
a great friend
to Rhona

YOUNG STAR: Like mother, like daughter.
Francesca follows in her mother's fairy
footsteps for a fancy dress party in 2003

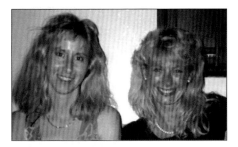 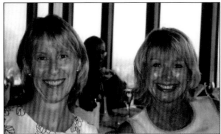

DOUBLE TAKE: Rhona with her friend Diane Bennett. Sixteen years separate these pictures

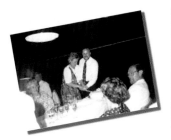 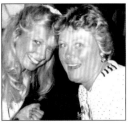 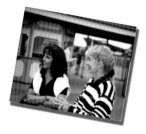

GREAT FRIENDS: From left, **John and Elizabeth Stones cut their cake on their 25th wedding anniversary, Rhona with Elizabeth in 1989 and Rhona with 'fairy friend' Laini in 1992**

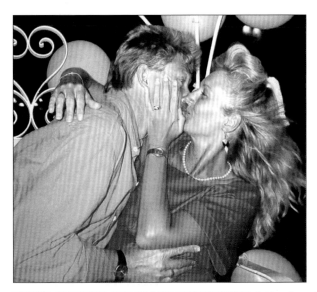 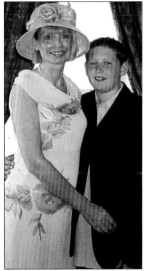

FRIEND, HUSBAND AND PILLAR OF STRENGTH: A kiss from David during a holiday in Mexico. Right, the chilling diagnosis that her cancer is terminal is seven days away for Rhona as she and her son Kristopher turn on the style for his godmother Becky's wedding

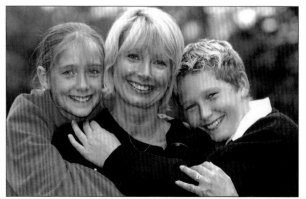

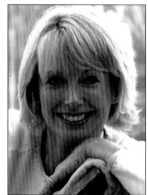

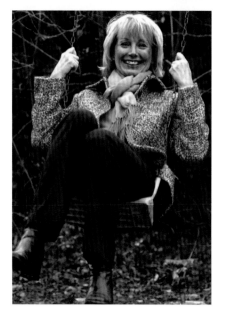

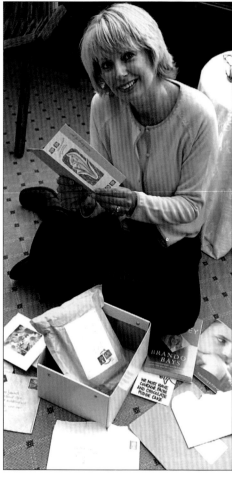

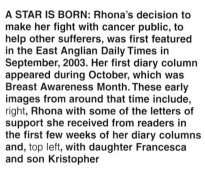

A STAR IS BORN: Rhona's decision to make her fight with cancer public, to help other sufferers, was first featured in the East Anglian Daily Times in September, 2003. Her first diary column appeared during October, which was Breast Awareness Month. These early images from around that time include, right, Rhona with some of the letters of support she received from readers in the first few weeks of her diary columns and, top left, with daughter Francesca and son Kristopher be the top cancer hospital in the country. It's got to the point where I'm embarrassed speaking to the secretary in the unit, saying: 'Hi, it's Rhona again, can you get someone to phone me?'."

(As told to Katy Edwards. Rhona was too tired to write her column herself this week.

A spokesperson at The Royal Marsden NHS Foundation Trust, said: "The Royal Marsden NHS Foundation Trust is very sorry to learn that Mrs Damant has been unhappy with some aspects of her care at the hospital.

"The trust has been making every effort to rearrange Mrs Damant's CT scan and it has now been rebooked for this week. Mrs Damant also has an appointment at the hospital this week when we will go over all aspects of her care, and do our best to redress any problems that have arisen. We shall also make a referral for further specialist symptom control")

May 10, 2004: *We all had such a brilliant time*

HI, its me again...See, I am still around! Sorry I was unable to write my diary last week but I am sure you all read what a nightmare I have had.

My tiredness and pain were at a level I have not experienced before and with that came a really poor level of concentration. Instead of writing a readable column it would have probably ended up like a script from *Bill and Ben* (yes, unfortunately I am that old and do remember them very well) - all "flobbalobbalob".

I am lucky that I had the backing of Katy last week. Unlike the pleas from my doctor and Macmillan nurse, the Marsden decided to respond to her call very quickly (I wonder why?!)

I had a phone call from the top professor and it seems that I will be under his care from now on. A CT scan and an appointment to see him was booked for last Wednesday but, guess what? It was cancelled due to the scanner breaking down and rebooked for Thursday, but at least that meant I would only have to have one needle as I would have my bone-drip at the same time.

I will now see the professor this Wednesday, together with a member of the palliative care team to talk me through symptom control. This will be the first time that I will have met them so I hope that it will be beneficial to me.

The power of a journalist can certainly make things happen but, unfortunately, most people don't have a "Katy" in their lives so will often accept what is thrown at them, believing it is their fate.

It is so wrong that this should be allowed to happen in the 21st Century. Being a cancer patient is not something you choose, nor can buying over-the-counter painkillers cure it, so we depend on qualified people to help make our lives as comfortable as possible; we should not have to fight for this. We might get the odd benefit like disabled parking and transport but the frightening life that goes with both primary and secondary cancer is not an enviable one.

We, along with our families and friends, live a stressful life; so for those whose hands we are in, please make our lives a little easier by taking some of that stress away, and not adding to it.

Having chemo could never be described as wonderful, but people can help to make the whole ordeal as pleasant as possible for you. This was my experience when I had all of my treatment first time round at Essex Rivers NHS Trust. All of the staff there were great in every way, so it just goes to show that the warm and caring approach can happen.

All of last week wasn't easy for any of us, but I'm happy that I got there in the end; at least I now have a chance of getting back on to the (chemotherapy) drug that I think might work for me. What I am trying to say is: everyone's life is worth fighting for, if you cannot do it yourself try to find someone who can help you do it. Life is far too sweet to give away.

I have now stepped off my soapbox!

A few months ago, Center Parcs at Elveden Forest arranged for the four of us to have a weekend there. Thankfully I was allowed to "up" my pain relief just before this break, which meant that me and my family were able to have the most brilliant time.

We have never been there before so didn't quite know what to expect, but what Center Parcs laid on for us was way above our expectations. We had the luxury of an executive, very new villa. A full grocery pack was waiting for us on our arrival, including pretty much everything we needed for our weekend. Bikes were booked for us (which was very amusing for all as I had not ridden a bike for 30 years, and it showed)! David and I had the luxury of the afternoon in the Aqua Sauna - a selection of themed baths, "multi-sensory showers" and reflexology footbaths which was so relaxing, my husband fell asleep - what an embarrassment!

Dinner that evening was at Huck's Diner. The waiter who served our table did not know we were on a special weekend but it was obvious from his wonderful manner and friendliness that it was just how he always is. As for my son saying that he was the best waiter that he has ever had, well that is the highest compliment ever awarded. So Aidan, thank you for giving us a great meal to remember.

The following day I had a deluxe manicure with a lady called Shelley. She also did

not know what was going on, and she too was so lovely. My nails are not the best anymore due to treatments over the years, but she gave me the loveliest nails I have ever had. The management must be very proud to have such great members of staff.

K and F had a go on the high ropes, which didn't do my heart much good, but they had great fun. Having started the weekend being just OK I certainly left, once again, feeling high up my adrenaline tree, but (and there is always a but, isn't there?) I have slept nonstop for the two days since coming back to a life that doesn't include a jacuzzi. So David, as I am unable to go out now for many lunches and am saving you LOTS of money can I have one in my bathroom just like I had at Elveden... please?

It seems that this week is one full of "thank yous" because here is another one. Just before we set off on our adventurous weekend, I received a beautiful bouquet from a family who live near Ipswich. The colours were gorgeous and, as they arrived in water, I was able to take them with me to Center Parcs. It always amazes me that people are so very kind as to actually take time out of their lives to do this for me. To that family, please can I say a huge THANK YOU.

I have had some more lovely letters sent on to me from Katy, they really do make my day. To those who have sent me addresses of places for healing and other helpful ideas I will next week, when I have more free time than I usually have, decide on things that I would like to do.

Francesca and her friend Irene are running in the Race for Life (for Cancer Research UK) on Sunday at Norwich. They both ran it together last year and they are doing it for me again this year. It was a very emotional event for me then and I know it will be the same if not worse for both David and myself this time. They won't be the fastest runners of the day, but does that matter? Just being able to watch my baby girl run along with her friend who I have watched grow up will be better than anything.

Well, I said two weeks ago that I would write and tell you all about our day recently with Anglia Television, but as I have managed to probably over fill my diary this time (again!) I don't think that it will be this week either, so read all about it next time...I hope!

Before I sign off, a few more "thank yous." Should my life not allow the Damant family to have another break or holiday together, can I just say that we will all be forever grateful to Katy for arranging this and to Center Parcs for their huge generosity in giving all of us a weekend that gave us good fun and quality time as a "normal" family again. I know none of us will ever forget it. The memories will always be with David and the children of absolute pure enjoyment, with me having a constant smile on my face, and for once, not letting myself feel tired.

Rhona x

May 17, 2004: *What a week of ups and downs*

I'M not very sure exactly where to start this week. Excuse me if it is all over the place, but you see today I had horrible news, and it has sent me into quite a daze.

You may remember me mentioning my great friends John and Elizabeth, who I have known for most of my life and who live in York. They have a son, Chris, and daughter, Becky, who is Kristopher's godmother. Chris, aged just 38, has just been diagnosed with quite a rare type of cancer that should only occur, apparently, in people over the age of 50. Chris has been a rugby player most of his life and played for a Yorkshire team for many years. He is very healthy, fit and mentally very strong, but

'I wish that I could give them all a cuddle'

when I phoned him, this strapping big lad had crumbled and become a sobbing, desperate, grief-stricken person. I spoke to him and his wife Liz but no amount of encouragement from me could stop him from thinking that his life had finished. All I can do for them is to be there at the end of a phone.

Unfortunately many miles separate us, and I wish more than anything that I could give them all a cuddle, but instead the best I can do is listen to the cries of a young couple whose perfect world has just fallen apart.

They will, in time, start to come to terms with and live with this thing, but at the moment Chris is insistent that future days will all be as black as this one, and refuses to believe what I say. So we have placed a bet on which one of us is right. At stake is one very expensive bottle of red wine, and I am determined that I will win! So there, Christopher Stones. Get your money out!

Now then, the good old Marsden! I had my CT scan and bone-drip last week (huge ouch) and I was also able to see a doctor I have met before and who has always been very nice. She was the person to break the

47

news to me in January about my heart and lungs. Although I previously said that I did not want to have any further chemo, with all the pain and the feeling of starting to lose my fight a little, chemo has reappeared on my wish list, but only providing that it is a non hair-losing one (see, I don't ask for much!).

I asked about having Capecitobine again (my last wonder-chemo tablet), so was surprised the treatment they were considering wasn't chemo but a hormone drug called Letrozole. This is for post-menopausal women, which, after almost five years of Tamoxifen, seemed to be the drug for me.

When I was told of all the benefits, I felt I was on the way forward again. The doctor prescribed it, David collected it from the pharmacy and I was ready to start taking my new lease of life the following day.

BUT THEN, the doctor returned and told me that a blood count of 100 is needed to start the tablets and mine was 98. So you've guessed it - I am sitting at home with very expensive drugs which I can only look at.

I am both annoyed and upset that I was told of all the benefits and how good they would be for me before they checked my blood count to see whether or not I was suitable.

I was supposed to return to the hospital on Wednesday for a bone scan, my CT and blood results, and have consultations with the 'Big Man' and the radiotherapy team, as it would seem that my main pain is coming from my ribs.

But on Tuesday, just as I was about to start a busy day of shopping and lunch, I became rather sick very quickly. I knew that I would be unable to make the trip to London the following morning at 5.30am, so had to cancel all my appointments. Luckily, it has all been all rearranged for next Wednesday.

David did ring the doctor up today and asked her to phone me with the results from last week's scan, as to wait for another week would just pull my mind to bits.

I knew what I wanted to ask and although my tummy was knotted with anxiety, I felt strong enough to take the news. When the call finally came, all my questions completely disappeared from mind when she said that it all looked the same as last time.

I felt jubilant initially, but then I asked about my cough, which is beginning to sound like the one I had this time last year and was told was a viral infection. Oh and as for my new drug, it is still a no-no.

My cough, I know, is not viral, because it is progressing in the same way as the last time, when it got to the stage of me being unable to speak more than three words in a row and having such awful coughing attacks that I was sick. I have decided that the only thing certain from that conversation is that I must continue looking at the new drugs, just wishing that I could feel the benefits.

My beautiful little girl and her life-long friend Irene ran the Race for Life last Sunday, on what was the most horrible of days in Norwich. Anglia Television covered the race to feature in the documentary. Francesca now believes herself to be rather famous having been seen on TV and written about in the EADT in the same week.

When Francesca and Irene ran the race last year, I really did not believe that I would be around to see them both do it again this year. I may have a thinner face with rather becoming black circles under my eyes and more weight from my liver than I would actually like, but there I was, emotional, but also excited about these two little people running for breast cancer.

They both ran the whole circuit. Francesca came in with a time of 29 minutes 18 seconds, with Irene not far behind, and both girls beat their times from last year. Francesca is also running another race in June with some of her school friends. It is very hard to put into words how proud I feel that so many of them are doing this with me in mind.

So just for that, when I return as a fairy, I will make sure you will all be on my good fairy list!

As many of you will have read on the front page of *Health*, Katy is doing a driving challenge in June, which I hope I will be able to attend. It was so lovely being allowed to choose the charity.

Obviously I thought that Breakthrough Breast Cancer should be "it" as we know that the money raised will be kept and used locally.

Well, sorry Anglia Television, once again I've written too much. I promise that I will write about our brilliant day next week!

Rhona x

May 24, 2004: *A wonder drug - and fighting again*

GUESS who is on a new lease of life?... ME! Almost one year after re-diagnosis (June 6, 2003) - a year of living with terminal cancer - I have been given the gift of being allowed to go back on my "wonder drug" Capecitabine.

There have been no promises made of it restraining the cancer, as it did so magically last year, but I am determined it will.

I at last saw Professor Smith at the Marsden on Wednesday. It was very nice that we could understand each other, as he is Scottish and his accent is very similar to my Northern Irish accent; even after 26 years living in England, I still have problems with people understanding me ... even my husband!

I was unable to go on the hormone drug recommended two weeks ago as it appeared my ovaries were still trying to work; as my body won't let them, however, taking those tablets means I would actually get worse instead of better. By then it didn't matter too much as it was the chemo drug that I really wanted and, by that stage, I had it back in my life again. I asked if I could go on tablets for my bones instead of having this much-too-frequent drip. The answer was no.

I quickly asked if I could have it closer to home instead, at Colchester, for example, and, much to my amazement, I could. Talk about my lucky day!

The hospitals will now work together on my treatment so "hi ho", it's off to Colchester I go ... what a luxury, just 20 minutes up the road instead of three hours. With all of this happening I now feel like I used to and I am going to love

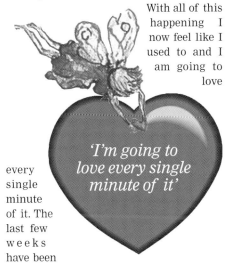

'I'm going to love every single minute of it'

every single minute of it. The last few weeks have been hard, as I could just not accept that the fight in me was going and I was getting too tired to get it back. I was aware that I needed some extra help for me to stay in this battle and now I have it.

It would have been my mum's birthday on my appointment day, and now the question

49

is: Was this her present to me or did my wishes come true due to a certain lady called Katy Edwards?

Who knows, but either way I have been given yet another chance to get my combat gear on again! I am going to London tomorrow to hear the results of my bone scan.

In the past couple of weeks, the pain in my legs, arms and hands has been excruciating; it feels like every bone has been broken. The cause of this is either that my oestrogen level has fallen too low, or that the cancer is back on its hike again - all will be revealed on Tuesday!

'If a goal is reached, I make another one'

With the good, came the bad and, even worse, the embarrassing! The bad was that my last good vein joined the other disobedient mob so I have to make up my mind soon on whether I have the permanent line under my chest or opt for the very high risk of using my right arm.

My lymph nodes were highly diseased during round one, which meant having over 20 removed when I had my mastectomy. Any damage to my arm or hand on that side could lead to lymphodema (I will explain more about this next week), which would mean refraining from having needles.

To most, it would seem that I am being extremely stupid for even thinking about it but then there is also my fear of having further surgery, so it is a difficult choice.

The embarrassment was my dosage of tablets. When I went on this chemo last year I had lost quite a lot of weight and was just seven stone. This year I am heavier, and now have the extra bonus of a swollen liver.

I previously took six tablets a day but now take twelve. When I went to take them on the first night I thought that the prescribed dose was wrong and phoned the hospital, only to be told the dosage was calculated on weight. It would seem this was my answer... the pleasure of having cancer has turned me into a "pear".

Goals are a big part of my life and will continue to be so; as soon as one is reached I make another one.

Francesca has just completed two for me, with the "Race for Life" and by reaching her teens (madness I know, to wish a teenager upon myself but I needed to see my baby do it).

The love of her life (and just about the rest of the female world) is Jonny Wilkinson. I spent several weeks trying to have a card sent to her from this "fit number 10" but was unsuccessful.

Her mum couldn't do it but Katy did, so, on May 15, my daughter became one of the more unusual teenagers by being happy! What would I do without a "Katy" in my life?

Anglia News featured part of my documentary recently. For those who watched it I hope it gave you more of an insight into the Damant family. It is a very true picture.

We had a VIP day to the Anglia Television studios in Norwich last month. We started off with a great lunch at Tony's house (my personal cameraman!) then a studio tour.

We met David Jennings, editor for *Anglia News East*, who planned an exciting day for the children and an interesting one for David and myself. We saw how the news goes from the planning stage right through to transmission.

I also saw my documentary for the first

time. It was in different sequences, but I had to ask not to see some as K & F were watching.

There are a few sensitive issues and, although one day they will see them, I don't think the time is right just yet.

The making of this true story can be difficult for all of us at times but I have always been very fortunate to have such a caring team behind me, including someone who I have not mentioned before, Mike Talbot.

The editor is Johnny Moore who, up until then, I hadn't met. I must admit I felt a little anxious meeting someone with his high reputation and status but what a lovely person he was. Now that I have met Johnny (who is very much younger than I anticipated) I will always feel happier knowing, whether I see it or not, that this will be my story filmed, written and produced by people who I trust so much that I have given them access into my family life.

I hope that this, just like this diary you are reading, will in time be that film that I couldn't find ... to show all sides of cancer, good and bad.

Rhona x

May 31, 2004: *Bad news has sent me tumbling down*

Isn't life like a game of snakes and ladders? One throw of a dice has you climbing to the top of the ladder and then the next throw has you tumbling back down again; often even further down than you had started out.

No one can ever make themselves throw that six, just the same as no matter how many portions of fruit and vegetables we have a day, we have no guarantee of being the healthiest people around.

Our lives often seem to be beyond our control through no fault of our own, just like the dice : "whatever will be, will be".

Last week I climbed the tallest ladder, but this week it was time for the poisonous snake. May 19 brought me the magic of my wonder drug and then, six days later, came the news that my cancer had spread to my legs, arms and also, surprisingly, my skull.

Deep down, I knew that this was going to be the case as there was absolutely no way in this world my pain could have been associated with a low level of oestrogen. The lack of this hormone, I imagine, does create much pain; but to be woken up several times a night, feeling that my legs and arms had been crushed to the point of every bone being broken did not sound like a hormonal problem to me.

It didn't matter how mentally ready I was for this news, the day following these unwanted results sent me to the land of aliens and tears.

My idea of bone cancer has never included my skull. Brain tumours are naturally associated with cancer, but not once have I ever thought it would affect my skull. When you read the meaning of skull in the dictionary, it quotes "bony case of the brain, the bones of the head"; there is my answer...the skull is bone.

The quote goes on to mention "Crossbones: emblem of death, having two thighbones crossed". The thighbone is the leg above the knee - where do you think my cancer has just moved to ...my upper leg! I have never thought of bone cancer as a "killer" (in future I will sit with my legs uncrossed as I don't want to think of myself as the "emblem of death").

I have decided not to ask too many questions about anything at this stage - I am sure I could quite easily make myself believe that I have every symptom possible. The not knowing is better for me right now, as my

51

mind has gone into temporary emotional turmoil and until I can think straight again, I don't want, or in fact need, those answers.

Just after I had the results I saw a consultant radiotherapist, who was great. In her words, there were too many "hot spots", otherwise known as cancer to you and me! As luck would have it, they had quite a free day, so a slot was found to allow me to have a huge blast (of radiotherapy) within an hour.

I had three people marking me up with black pen - instead of those little needle dots, which I don't care for too much. As the pain in my ribs covers a large region, it was decided that I would show them exactly where it hurts most so that this whole area could be included in the "blast". I think it took them quite by surprise as they started off with a small square but then had to go to the largest.

Calculation of the dose was completed quite quickly, so off I went to a room I have come to know extremely well. I had about five minutes of what is hoped will be my new painkiller and was told that skin discomfort would be rather painful as they had used a piece of equipment that sat almost on top of the skin, rather than the usual longer distance away.

Other side-effects were mentioned too, such as tiredness and nausea, due to the close proximity of the treatment to my liver.

It wasn't until I arrived back home that I realised how stupid my rib area looked; a huge black square containing 17 dots, which could easily pass as a page from a children's drawing book!

I have been told that it might take two weeks to see any evidence of the effects of the radiotherapy and that, in the meantime, I have to be very careful with that side, rubbing it with E45 cream.

Those times when David and I used to go to London for the day, whenever I had clinic appointments, now seem like part of anoth-er life. We would shop...actually no, I would shop and he would stand outside with that look that only men can master when their partner is running riot inside with a cheque book! We would then go to our favourite restaurant, enjoy our lunch, which always included a bottle of wine, then off to the Marsden, followed by a walk down Kings Road and David's fear of getting too close to the Pier (my all-time favourite shop) before starting for home.

Now lunch is a sandwich at outpatients (made by the ladies from the Friends of the Marsden, who can be quite frightening!) and tea from a plastic cup, which tastes good all the same.

The funny thing is, we don't remember our last proper lunch, I wonder how we would have coped with it had we known what was in store for us all?

On Tuesday, we did wonder about going out for lunch again, as we had finished so early, but we both knew that the scan results would take the pleasure away for us.

On a day like this we are often unable to talk very much. We probably look like that long-married couple who have nothing to say to one another!

I noticed one couple snapping at each other at the hospital; the lady wouldn't let her husband see any of her paperwork. It turned out she had just been diagnosed. David reminded me of how emotional that day had been for us - do you know, for the first time, I realised that I never once thought of how he was feeling on that Wednesday morning in August 1999 when I told him over the phone that we had to go to hospital to see the oncologist.

Looking back, I behaved exactly like this lady who, in her mind, had been given a death sentence and whose life would change forever.

Mine did, hers will, and for all those one-in-three people who become cancer victims, life will never again be the same as it was before the fateful diagnosis day.

Katy always keeps my letters until a little pile has appeared, then she posts them off to me and I have the excitement of a child opening a present as I sit down with a cup of tea and read them.

My memory box is getting larger as time goes on and every one I get is read and re-read, each is so special to me. It has amazed me just how many people have taken such an interest in my story.

'It is my family and friends who deserve all the praise'

Several years ago in one of the Sunday papers a similar story was featured every few months. My friend Laini and I would read, cry, talk and follow it, and to this day, we have never forgotten it. The lady in question did eventually die, leaving three very small children.

A few years later a follow-up story was written about her husband and how he coped being a single dad - he did remarry again and created a new life for himself, so happiness for him did follow the sadness.

From all my letters the words "brave, inspirational, courageous and admirable" are often used, but I am sorry to say I am really none of those things - it is my family and friends who deserve all those words and more. I can sleep a lot, and therefore be else-where, but it is those around me, especially David and the children, who have to watch someone who was once a busy mum and wife turn into a slow, sleepy, sore, and at times, emotional nightmare.

I would like to say from Francesca and myself a heartfelt thank you to a very generous and kind man - someone who can only be described as one of the world's true gentlemen - from Woodbridge for sending sponsorship money for the "Race For Life", which Francesca will run again in June.

I have rarely seen my daughter as over-come as she was when we received the cheque this week. Both of us could not believe how kind you were, the money you sent will go to Cancer Research UK, which funds vital research into all forms of can-cer. I know, throughout her life, Francesca will always remember you as this lovely man who she will never know but who cared enough to sponsor her. Thank you.

I had wanted to talk about other things this week, but I'm afraid the mass destruc-tion of my healthy cells has been my major talking point, but then that is all part of a cancer diary... unfortunately.

Rhona x

June 7, 2004: *Feeling fired up to play taxi driver*

THIS cancer thing is beginning to con-fuse me quite a lot now. Last week when I was writing my diary, I had just been given the news about the latest naughty cell invasion, and life was not look-ing good.

One week later, I feel great!

Thankfully, this latest burst of energy arrived in time for half term, which meant for the first time in ages during K & F's hol-idays I have felt a "proper" mum. I have been given the chance once again to play taxi driver. And I have loved every minute of it!

On one of the days, we went to All Fired Up, in Ipswich, a favourite school holiday haunt for us for some time now. Kristopher's best friend Jonno teams up with us every time and this was no exception. We used to all sit together, but now the boys always are the two in the corner pretending not to be with anyone!

The bank has been broken, the sun hasn't shined, but it's been great, unlike past years, when it has been a case of, "oh no, not another half term".

I'm not sure what exactly has happened to make me return to the "good life". Is it the chemo working, or maybe just knowing that I'm back on my wonder drug. Then again, it could be the fact that I have now returned to Colchester for my treatment and am suddenly a person with a name again, rather than being a six-figure number in London. Whatever it is, it is definitely working and that is enough for me.

Everything has happened very quickly with my return to Colchester. I had my first visit last Tuesday and start my treatment on Wednesday. The nurse who was unlucky enough to know me first time round is still there. He remembered me through my fear of needles, or so he said, but I think it was due to the fact that I always turned up late as high as a kite from valium and managed to trip over the same step. Few people are likely to have made an entrance like that too often.

They will probably never own up that they had a celebration drink when I left after my last treatment in December 1999, followed by a commiseration drink when "it" returned!

When I was waiting for my appointment I met a lady who reads my column. We had quite a lengthy chat, which was lovely because if she didn't read the diary, we would never have met. We both wondered why it was that in hospital waiting rooms we get comfy chairs, but then, when it is nearly time for our appointment, we have to move to a hard seat. Is it to wake us all up? I wish they would leave us in comfort for a little while longer.

Exactly four years ago I had a party for all my friends, as I was then officially free from cancer. It doesn't feel as if 1465 days have passed since that night, when I dined on champagne.

My invitations read: "It was a battle fought and won" and I believed it to be true. Life should then have gone back to normality, of sorts. But, of course, it didn't. I would do absolutely anything in this world to be able to turn the clock back to that night of sheer indulgence and happiness - why did it all have to go so very wrong?

I, like most other people, have had moments in life where the air has turned blue. I'm thinking of when I hid under Kristopher's bed to get a few minutes' peace from noisy toddlers, but did I really deserve all this? Even my Macmillan nurse said I could get a place in the *Guinness Book of Records* for the amount of cancer in my body!

One of my all-time favourite songs is by Queen. Some lines have special meanings for me: "What is this thing that builds our dreams yet slips away from us? It's all decided for us. This world has only one sweet moment set aside for us."

The title is *Who Wants to Live Forever?* I felt the words had a special something ever since I first heard it. It is all very poignant to me now, but if it meant always being with my children, then yes, I would want to live forever.

Recently, I touched a little on lymphoedema, as the reason why I really should not have any treatment on my right arm. During my mastectomy, many lymph nodes were also removed due to them also being diseased. Lymph is a colourless fluid that forms in the tissues of the body. It normally drains back into the blood through the lymphatic system. Lymph nodes or glands act as filters removing dead or abnormal cells and bacteria.

Oedema means swelling, so lymphoedema means swelling in the tissues below the skin when lymph can't drain properly. This can happen if nodes are reduced or scarred after surgery or treatment, which results in less effective drainage from fluid in the affected area of the body.

I did escape this, but there are certain precautions that people at risk can take to avoid overloading the remaining lymph drainage routes.

Infection and inflammation can be caused by cuts and scratches not cleaned properly; injections, blood tests and blood pressure should be avoided if possible as should extremes of temperature. Exercise is good for the drainage system, but that arm should not be used for pushing, lifting and heavy shopping.

The principal treatment is usually wearing a specially designed elastic support sleeve or stocking, which are just so gorgeous. Yes, I have been known to wear one from time to time but, believe me, it does work!

So, that ends another week of the highs, the lows and the other side of cancer - when the lymph nodes decide to misbehave!

Rhona x

June 14, 2004: *What a difference a year makes*

EXACTLY one year ago I was an inpatient at the Marsden and felt I was on the outside of a window looking in. I had absolutely no control over my life.

Looking back, I find it difficult believing that person could really have been me.

If I turned the clock back, I would now be in the middle of my worst-ever nightmare, having a treatment with the delightful name of "intra fecal".

It could only be carried out by specialised staff and only on one particular ward. I had to lie on my back, curled up with the doctor behind me. A needle was then inserted into the fluid surrounding the spinal cord. From this, a lumbar puncture was carried out and with the needle still in place chemo was then injected, which seemed to take forever.

Quite a large dressing covered the needle entry point. I had to remain on my back for two hours with my blood pressure taken quite frequently. I never actually felt ill afterwards but my head always felt as if it was stuffed with cotton wool.

Things always seem to happen to me that never happen to other people and this was no exception. During my first experience of this ghastly, horrible, true-life bad dream, the fire alarm went off, which meant the fire brigade had to come out. Every time I had this treatment, supper would always arrive at the same time. Two hours later it would still be at the end of my bed. It looked so disgusting even a hungry stray animal wouldn't have sniffed at it twice!

After two hours of lying flat, they had another little shock treatment in store for me - a drug called Zoladex, used in women who have breast cancers that are sensitive to oestrogen. It may feel uncomfortable to most people but with my needle phobia it was fearsome!

It is an implant injection under the skin of the stomach, intended to switch off oestrogen production from the ovaries (and therefore help control the cancer). My eyes were tightly closed when they gave it to me, so it felt like a very sharp tiny flat spoon being shot into my stomach, but it was actually a syringe and needle. I have heard peo-

55

ple talk about this drug being used for other problems, so it would seem a good all-rounder but I wouldn't classify it among my favourites!

Needles, drugs, tests, sickness; but worst of all, doctors constantly being brought in to look at me, making me feel like part of a freak show. I just happened to be that unfortunate person, with such a huge amount of cancer, the professor liked to show me off.

All this made for the worst week in my entire life. At that stage, it looked unlikely the hospital would allow me to go to Australia. The best I could hope for was to still be around for the school holidays. The outlook was so gloomy; every night when I went to sleep in the little room on the ward, I made sure I kept my door wide open...just in case.

But that has all been in the past, I made it through the hot summer, and of course Australia, then Kristopher's birthday, followed by Francesca's entrance into teenage life.

My cancer is now even worse (I can't imagine what all the student doctors would think of me now if they saw me, maybe my files would have me down as an alien) but I'm still here and hopefully about to see another summer through.

One of my main goals was to see my daughter start upper school this September, as that to me is the beginning of her adult life. My wish list is as long as it ever has been, but I still am determined to visit Bath, have my hot air balloon trip with my family, show my children where their grandma (my mum) is buried in Ireland, and see my book of my weekly diaries in print.

So will I achieve it? Of course I will!

Francesca is counting down her last few weeks at Stoke by Nayland Middle School. Even though I want to see her at Sudbury Upper, her last day will be a tearful one for me. I don't want to have to let go of her being a child but it is the right time for her to step forward into the next stage of her life.

Since my re-diagnosis, the teachers and office staff have comforted my children and treated me with the dignity a cancer sufferer hopes for.

Each year they have a fundraising week with the children choosing a charity. This year's is Suffolk Breakthrough Breast Cancer. It is such a privilege for me to think the children and staff will be competing in all sorts of weird and wonderful ideas, to raise as much money as possible for breast cancer.

Their charity last year was the air ambulance, but as I was in hospital that week, my two were allowed to also do their own fundraising for the Marsden and raised more than £200. Good luck Stoke, enjoy every minute of it, but don't forget to collect those pennies at the end.

'We laughed our way back to the hospital'

I had my first treatment at Colchester on Tuesday. I can't say that I enjoyed every minute of it, but it wasn't anything like my London trips.

My friend Mary collected me at 10.30am and for the next hour we managed to do the "girly" thing of trying on too many dresses in town. By the time we had laughed our way back to hospital I had completely forgotten to take my "calm-me-down" tablet, which meant that, for the first time ever, I did not fall over that same step that always used to trip me up.

The cannula went into my wrist first time, the doctor saw me, my chemo was prescribed and at 4.30pm I went home, so how could anyone complain about that day?

My chemo dosage has been increased and has been approved by the Marsden. I didn't ask why because I can only think of one explanation and I'm not very keen on hearing that right now.

When I got home, my wrist was very swollen and sore so I think my vein has been blown (yet again!) but I expect I can cope with that one too! I'm off to take some of my 27 daily tablets, so speak to you next week,

Rhona x

June 21, 2004: *Feeling tired after a rocking week*

DUE to a busy week, I am now feeling very tired. (Reminder to myself; take at least one day off to rest).

It all kicked off last Saturday, when David, Francesca and myself (Kristopher is definitely now a teenager, as sleep seems to be more important than anything) went to watch Katy (Edwards) do her driving challenge. Of course, being an outside event, the good old English weather decided it just had to be on what was about the worst day for months. We eventually found one another (what would we do without mobile phones?) and managed to get a quick photograph together before the black cloud appeared.

It was very difficult to watch Katy driving as most of the vehicles were in a security zone, quite a distance away from the spectators - and from the husbands who all seemed to be very amazed to see those women driving just perfectly!

Katy has raised nearly £1,500, which, initially, I didn't think would be possible. But it has all been down to the generosity of EADT readers. What can be said, but a huge THANK YOU!

Her husband was telling us that when they both went to the recent Will Young concert in Ipswich, people were actually putting money into Katy's hand. What wonderful people you all are.

Francesca's school, Stoke By Nayland Middle School, has also been having fun (except I'm not so sure that the teachers would agree) with their fundraising for the same charity - Suffolk Breakthrough Breast Cancer. And just like Katy, they have been raising an unbelievable daily amount.

Wednesday was the media day so, naturally, the mother was there too. Events have been taking place both indoors and out. In all honesty, the teachers should be given a week of compassionate leave for what they have had to do.

As Mrs Yallop, my mentor for activities week, said: "They don't tell you anything like this in teacher training!"

The main event that I watched was "I'm a teacher, get me out of here". If it had been me, I'm afraid I would have gone!

Male teachers had their legs waxed. Ouch, ouch, ouch! Added to that was: applebobbing in a bowl of cream and baked beans, drinking a glass of tomato ketchup and Tabasco sauce - just how bad is that? dancing in front of cool pupils, all with multi-coloured hair for bad hair day, 10 marshmallows in a mouth in 10 seconds, identifying objects in dog food, with the grand finale of cream pies for those poor unsuspecting teachers!

Totals will not be known until later in the week as money is still coming in. Children, staff, parents and friends of the school should all feel so proud of themselves for giving so generously to the UK's leading breast care cancer charity, committed to research and raising awareness. The money will be kept in our local area, which is another good thing. There is one "but" - it's just that I wish more than anything that it wasn't me that has brought all of this about.

As well as returning to my life of lunches I also had the great opportunity of watching Elton John in concert at Portman Road. He was absolutely superb.

With the good, however, also comes the embarrassing - my friend LW. Our seats were close to the front and Mrs W decided to join a gentleman who was swaying/dancing to the music all on his lonesome. Thankfully, soon after that, EJ sang one of his great oldies, so we were all on our feet, but it made it a memorable night for her poor husband and friends who could only watch her in disbelief. We always had this feeling that we would grow old disgracefully, well that's it then, we have started!

My night of pure enjoyment came as a present from one very lovely lady, Teresa Durling. Without her, it would have been a night of TV and (I am ashamed to admit) *Big Brother*. Instead, five of us had an evening of fun, memories, and laughter. Is there any other way of living life? So Teresa I grant you now a place on my lovely fairy list.

A concert like that should be a special evening for all, but as is always the way, there is often one who has to spoil it for everyone else and I'm afraid to say this was no exception. Just in front of us, a very large gentleman in a very colourful shirt decided it was his right to threaten the young lad sitting directly behind him. This lad and his girlfriend couldn't see as the large man's smaller friend was standing on his seat.

As we were near the front we could all watch Sir Elton very well without even having to look at the screens but this person had to ruin everyone's view with his stupid behaviour. He still didn't get down from his seat for some time even after one of the stewards had come over. It is such a shame that when people go out for a night to leave all their troubles behind them for just a short time, there is always someone with that self-centred air, not giving a thought to other people. Just why do they feel the need to be like this?

Now on my second session of chemo, I have started to notice the strength going in my hair. The same thing happened exactly one year ago - both on Monday, June 16, 2003 and on Wednesday, June 16, 2004 - my shoulder-length hair became a very short bob.

I was very hesitant to go that short this time but I knew it was the right thing to do as after only five weeks on chemo my hair was becoming very wispy. In my beloved husband's words: "It was doing nothing for you". Why can't men be nice about the truth? Couldn't he have just said something like: "Maybe it's time for a change"? Obviously it's a bloke thing to tell it like it is!

Just before I go, I would like to share with you a comment made to me within minutes of meeting someone who I hadn't seen for a year.

Stupidly, I expected her to greet me with something like "Hi how are you?" How wrong I was. She said: "Aren't you embarrassed you are still alive? After all, a year ago, you thought that you were going to die soon, but you are STILL here!"

So, given that I really should have died long ago, perhaps I should now hibernate until the time comes when I am about to take my last breath and then make an appearance again.

It upsets me that someone could think that. I just hope that other people aren't thinking the same!

Rhona x

58

June 28, 2004: *A big thank you to the fundraisers*

ALL of last week my daughter's school, Stoke By Nayland Middle School, held an activities charity week in aid of Suffolk Breakthrough Breast Cancer.

The children had to think up a list of events. They weren't allowed to do a lot of things they'd done in past years, such as contact sports between teachers and children, but they still managed a good week.

Everyday the pupils baked and sold cakes in the tuck shop, raising huge amounts of money. For most of the week the teachers had a dreadful time. "I'm a Teacher Get Me Out of Here" was hilarious - I watched as one of the male teachers had his legs waxed, another had to plunge his hands into dog food, another was apple bobbing into a dish of cream and baked beans and then there was the 10 marshmallows into the mouth in 10 seconds. You name it, everything revolting those children could think of, they made their teachers do it!

And, I am ashamed to say my own daughter, Francesca, was one of the initiators. It was her who thought up the baked beans.

A netball match between teachers and children was also a hit, with girls dressed as fairies and teachers as skater boys. The teachers got their own back, winning 7-6.

Then there was "Distraction", where teachers had to answer questions whilst being shot by water pistols, pupils vs teachers rounders, teachers' "*Millionaire*", pupils' "*Blind Date*", tug of war, "*Pop Idol*", a *Mission Impossible* assault course, air guitar competition, remote control lorry challenge, sponge the teachers. The list goes on.

Those poor teachers definitely deserve a medal. The parents also helped raise a huge amount of money. Francesca managed to raise £150 on her own. The school hasn't got a final total yet as money is still coming in but it promises to be huge. People have gone to so much effort - in Francesca's words: "every little helps". It will all go towards fighting one of the biggest killers and, of course, the money raised will stay in Suffolk.

So I would like to say a big thank you to all the staff, pupils, parents and friends who have done their bit.

Other events of the week: I backed my car into a brick wall and banged my head really badly on the headrest. I think I must have dislodged the tumour in my brain. You wouldn't believe the things I've done.

The other day I was supposed to be going to Hintlesham Hall with my friend. I got up, got in the shower, rushed downstairs, put the kettle on, came up to dry my hair, only to realise after drying it for a few minutes that I hadn't actually washed it.

Then I came downstairs, picked up the lemonade thinking it was the kettle and filled my teacup. Then, I went upstairs again and got dressed - into my nightdress.

It's been an absolute joke of a week. It didn't stop there. I filled a pint with orange juice and dropped it all over our cream carpet. I hadn't bothered to shut my car roof properly so all that rain went into the car. I put the car through the car wash but hadn't taken my aerial off, so of course that

'You wouldn't believe the things I've done'

snapped off. This has all been since I bumped my head. It has just been the most ridiculous week of my life.

I've got a scan coming up in a couple of weeks so we'll see then if I'm right about the tumour.

Rhona x

July 5, 2004: *Thanks girls, you make me feel so proud*

THANKFULLY, it hasn't been such a daft week, mentally, for me, except that I did manage to pour hot water on to my cornflakes instead of in my tea cup.

No doubt there will be further stories to tell you with the shenanigans of my now daft brain.

Now then, to the more important events of the past week: Race For Life.

We have been to Colchester and Norwich, so it was time to try the Bury race. Unlike the last race, the weather was just right for the runners. Francesca did her stuff again. This time she was joined by four other girls, two of them twins, with the lovely thing being they all had my name on their backs (Francesca almost slipped up, and was about to put me down "in memory"). Three of the girls have been friends of K & F for many years and I have watched them grow into beautiful teenagers. They were joined by the twins' older sister (just as gorgeous), who I only met on the day.

All I can say is what an honour it was to have someone run that distance for me without even really knowing me. The girls in question, who did me proud, were Laura Crofton, the twins Hannah, Hollie and older sister Nicola Jackson and, of course, not forgetting my own little 13-year-old. What more can I say girls, other than you were all absolutely fantastic. Thank you. Now start training for next year!

To my amazement I met someone else after the race who I didn't recognise at first, but later realised was one of the women from the vets we use. And guess what? My name was on her back as well. She is a lovely person and always takes time to ask how I am on our frequent visits when our little Westie decides to be as dysfunctional as the rest of the family.

Mine wasn't the only name that she had on her pink card, which, unfortunately for her, means she has been hit several times with this hateful "C" thing. Sadly, I didn't get the opportunity to sponsor her, so make sure you ask my husband next year.

The most important thing for most of those taking part is that all their sponsorship money is going to such a great charity. What makes it such fun day, however, is competing in such a wonderful atmosphere. At the end of the day, does it matter what time people run or walk it in? I imagine the most satisfying feeling would be just finishing at all.

I have just had my second visit to Colchester for my bone-drip and have been prescribed a new session of chemo. I don't know why I feel more at ease with my visits there rather than London.

Each time, as most of you will know, I always used to have to take a sedative to calm me down before my needle went in. But I have found this wasn't strictly necessary. I still do have to lie down but with the help of my friend Mary's hand (which I just about manage not to break every time) the job is done, and within minutes I am sitting back up again.

The nurse I had five years ago is still there (luckily for me) and, in David's words, probably has more experience than all of the Marsden day unit nurses put together -

60

for once in my life, I actually agree with my husband. Chris is the most gentle of nurses and would put anyone at their ease, which, with someone like me, must be the most difficult of jobs. Another nurse and myself decided between us which of my veins we should use, and hey presto! We got it right as Chris got the cannula in first time. My blood results have been better but still are high enough to be allowed another session of my good old wonder drug.

I do feel that it is working again for me but, of course, nothing will be known until I have further scans and tests to measure the size of all the tumours. As yet, I am not very sure when this will be, or even where, but I have been sent a follow-up appointment for the Marsden for September 1. Until I have the up-to-date results in my hands, I will continue to believe I am responding well.

Cancer is doing things to my body that I never thought would happen. It is so very different from the first time around, when I lost so much weight and resembled a skeleton. Due to the drugs, my liver, and the surgery from February, however, this time I have turned into the grandma from *The Kumars*. No I don't watch that, but I do know who she is from the adverts on television. There is pain in my legs and my stomach has grown to an enormous size!

My drugs mean I can now manage to forget the extent of the pain, but then I find myself hating my cancer even more for allowing me to become this horrible shape - huge around the middle, but very skinny in other places like my ankles and shoulders.

I never had to watch my weight in the past but even going without all yummy delights, my stomach is beginning to get me down.

For the first time ever, I am feeling my age, and am not as confident as I used to be when I am going out. Isn't it funny how we think of pain, weight loss and death when cancer is mentioned but you never hear how cancer can make your body resemble a drawing of a cartoon character who is both little and large.

I am just off now to add several inches to my stomach by having lunch with my friend Sue who, unfortunately, has her own health problems. Crazy as it sounds, it is great for us to get together as we are as scatty as one another.

Once again, we are going to Monks Eleigh, where we will spend hours trying to convince each other we need to spend our husbands' money by buying all the goodies for sale. As we both know only too well, we have to live for today and make the most of every tender moment.

Rhona x

July 12, 2004: *A day of true heartbreak*

THIS is going to be a very difficult diary for me to write this week, but equally I also think it may be hard for some of you to read. It has taken me several weeks to build up to the point of feeling that I can actually write it down, but I know it won't be all at once and will take me several hours to do it.

As I type, I am also telephoning several local shops, asking for prizes for the school as they are going to finish off their fund raising for Suffolk Breakthrough Breast Cancer by holding a raffle at the end of the week.

This all started with me ringing Ipswich Town Football Club to ask if it was possible to be given something. They came up trumps by donating a signed shirt. Next week I will publish (get me, with my new posh ways of writing!) the "roll of honour"

61

of all those who generously gave to Stoke by Nayland's chosen charity.

In the past week I have received a large envelope from Katy (at the EADT) with letters of support. With this she also included the many letters written when so many of you sent money for our local cancer charity.

Reading the letters brought many tears as I never thought I would be in a situation where so many people cared and prayed for me and my family. Thank you all so much for doing all this for me. But as I have passed the stage of any research ever helping me, I hope so much that in the future the money everyone has sent will help someone who lives in our neighbourhood to successfully fight this disease.

Before I start on the emotional side, I would just like to say to that "Ordinary Dad" out there, of course you can climb Sydney Harbour Bridge. I did it, as you said, which means you can too. Don't worry about the height, you are at the top before you know it. Just one word of advice; do not look up as you start the climb. Enjoy every minute of it. I would give anything to have the chance again.

Well here goes. As you know, last year on my birthday, I met our local vicar and chose my burial plot at Great Waldingfield church. A very strange thing happened a couple of months later. Someone said they had already put their name down for the same plot - and most of that row. This, to David and myself, was a case of déjà vu as one year after my dad's burial we had to lift and remove him to another plot. Apparently a baby had been buried there and when the parents returned after many years away, they found their unnamed area had my dad resting there.

I didn't mind where I went, as long as it was in the same area. In fact, I didn't even have to change at all but I thought it would be best to keep these people happy.

The children knew what had happened and were quite happy with it. However on a Saturday afternoon. Francesca said she wanted to go and visit her gramps (my dad) and bring fresh flowers.

When I lost my dad I went up each day at first, then it went to just a Sunday but since my own diagnosis I found it too close to home and ended up crying for days, meaning my visits are very few and far between now. But as my daughter wanted me to go, we went.

As soon as we reached the grave and put the flowers down, which started my tears straight away, she asked to see where I will go (oops, stop for a hankie break). We wandered quietly hand in hand, through the rambling greenery of the church until we reached the spot. It was there that my little girl said: "But mummy, you can't go there, because when I come up everyday to see you and do my homework, I can't sit on the little seat watching over you and be close to you". As you can imagine, the tears were running down both our faces as we stood together having a huge cuddle.

I asked her where she would like me to go, so we chose the plot together, right behind the church tower, close to a memorial bench where she can sit in shelter regardless of the weather and just be with her mum. We sat together for a couple of hours until we both knew it was time to go, and with that she has not spoken about it again. It was a

'The tears were running down both our faces'

62

day of true heartbreak for me, and I seemed to remain in tears for the next few days.

When I felt that I was strong enough to do it I met with the vicar and we booked my new place. During the same week two very strange things happened.

The first was when a very close friend of ours announced she was pregnant. Now, there are other babies entering this world who I hope to meet on their arrival. But with his baby my immediate thought was "That is it, that will be my day to leave, one new life and one departed one."

Thankfully, our friends do not live close to me, as I would find it hard to continually share their excitement, but I can at least, always manage it on the phone or on the odd meeting.

The day following this news came another shock to my old brain. I was sitting in the conservatory on what was actually a sunny day and for the first time in 14 years of sitting on that seat, the sun beamed through the windows in the shape of a cross. I am sure I have been told I am now on my final road and with that I need to stay as stress-free as I can and enjoy every possible moment.

Most mums wouldn't even start to think of their daughter's wedding when she had just turned 13, but I need to know that I have arranged as much as possible before it is too late. That is why I have handed over my little precious to one of my closest and best friends to help her have the wedding her mum would have wanted for her, and with my friend being there with her during this stage of her life, I know that dream will be achieved. But, unfortunately for David, Francesca has said they will have to go to Italy, Paris or New York for that special dress. That's my girl. With Kristopher, I know that if he does make it into the RAF his life will be a good one, and should he ever decide to get married he will just let all the plans go over his head, like his dad did, and do his duty of just turning up on the day.

My biggest, and at the time unthinkable, goal last June was to see Francesca start her walk into adulthood at upper school in September. There have been many times when I thought it would never happen and I know many other people thought the same, but I am now only eight weeks away from this, and have just been with her on the open night, met her year tutor and picked up the uniform. When she tried it all on, I knew I have done my job.

Just before I go, Francesca asked me during the week the question I have been dreading: "Mum how many months do you have left?" My stomach went into knots, I felt sick, started to stumble on my words. By this time she was getting highly frustrated, so the outburst came: "For goodness' sake mum, it is a simple question, how many months do you have left before you can change your mobile phone, as I am sick of mine and I would like you to get the one I want, so that maybe I can have yours - then you can have mine." And with that she charged out of the room, leaving one very relieved mum sitting with a smile on her face.

Rhona x

July 19, 2004: *Lacking motivation in this terrible week*

I HOPE I didn't upset too many people last week, when I spoke about my "emotional moments" (as I think I have said before, I used to have many "blonde moments" but now they have changed to the above).

I have had quite a few comments from my friends telling me never to do that to them

63

again! I had been unable to speak about it to most of my friends, due to the tear thing, so for most this was the first they knew about it.

I have had a terrible week, leading on from the previous week, when at first I thought I had picked up a stomach bug. I then went on to thinking that I might have had an overload to my system of chemo. I am now on 1000mg more each day than I was this time last year.

My weight did rocket up to what was unacceptable to me, as I am very small-boned, meaning that I had an increased dosage. But during the three sessions I have taken so far, I have plummeted again to my usual weight (my stomach still has me looking like Tweedledee and Dum, unfortunately) so by my reckoning I am now swallowing too much poison daily. With the gripping stomach cramps came extreme fatigue and huge lack of motivation to do absolutely anything.

All in all, I haven't had much quality of life recently. In two weeks, I have managed one lunch and a very "small" amount of shopping at Corncraft, one parents' evening with Francesca and one visit to a lovely couple I have met through my diary who live minutes away from me. (Isn't it strange how you can live somewhere for 14 years and never meet the people who live just around the corner?).

This can only mean one thing ... I am not very well. The one very exciting thing this week, however, was beginning to work on a cover for my book of diaries.

I can't believe that, in nine months, I am now only a few steps away from having that book, which have always felt is so desperately needed for those younger people facing the horrible diagnosis of cancer.

The proceeds from the book will go to various cancer charities but as yet I am not very sure of how many or, in fact, which ones will benefit.

During the time I have been writing this, I have contacted my Macmillan nurse about trying to get some sort of medicine for the now awful stomach cramps.

This, in turn, has had me speaking to my chemo nurse at Colchester, then back to my Macmillan nurse and, just now, I have had a phone call from my doctor to say that I have now got to go straight into Essex Rivers Jefferson Ward to have a full blood count taken, as I may be having a sort of chemo-induced infection, which is why I am feeling so dreadful.

I have tried every sort of persuasion technique that I know to stop me from going in and, of course, also having to have that dreaded needle ... but I am not getting away with any of it, so David is now on his way home to drive me there.

Francesca's mobile phone is arriving some time tomorrow, so in my mind that is a good enough reason to have to come home.

No one can know the amount of mumbled chit-chat about how she "JUST HAS TO HAVE" this particular phone, that I have had to endure over the past few days. I would never have put my dad through that. I do remember the time, however, when I was 14 and wanted some boots but, as it was only weeks away from my birthday, was told to wait until then. I decided on the silent treatment with him and only cooked him a pie for dinner (without anything else!).

After a few nights of this very burnt offering, I got my boots, so I suppose in my particular way I did exactly the same in my early teenage years!

Well, I'm off to change my bed linen, clean my bathroom and cooker before David comes back. He gets so annoyed with me when I have to clean things before I go on holiday or, in this case, hospital.

He can't understand why I have to do it but I know that all the girls out there will know exactly what I am talking about. I think it is just implanted in our brains that we need a clean house to come back to, whatever the reason!

Its now Thursday, July 15, at 5.25pm and I am off to face an evening I don't care for much at all. The funny thing is I was meant to go to the Marsden today to see my eye consultant (see...eye, that's quite a clever one for me at this moment in time, when I don't seem to have much of a sense of humour) but felt so unwell I had to cancel it.

Here I am, several hours later, going to hospital anyway. What a world, eh? David is doing his pacing thing now, so fingers crossed that all goes well.

Rhona x

July 26, 2004: *Thoughts of dying always on my mind*

I'M still not quite feeling myself (back in Ireland, they would say, "so now tell me, if you're not feeling yourself, who would you be then?").

In six days I have managed to acquire two nice new bruises, one on my wrist and one on the back of my hand, really ugly!

I did spend some time in hospital. Actually, in hindsight, I should have stayed there much longer, but I had to be at home all of Friday to take delivery of that much-wanted mobile phone. When Francesca told me the reason for wanting it, I could understand why. She wanted to take photos of her friends on her last day at middle school, as most of her peer group will go on to Great Cornard Upper, whereas she and just a handful of others are going to Sudbury. If it had been me, I would have brought a camera but then I am 43 and not 13!

Kristopher also had a discovery day and therefore needed a packed lunch - another reason for me to get back home - so very late that evening we came home to a nice clean house! David still can't believe why I went into a spring cleaning mode in the half hour before I went to hospital but my friends understand - in fact, most of them are doing that right now, before they depart on their holidays.

All this just goes to show that life can't stop when you are a mum with terminal cancer!

I think a lot of the hesitation of not wanting to go on to a ward was down to that fear of the unknown.

More and more over the past couple of months, over silly little things, I have found myself acting not at all in the mature adult way I should.

This was one evening like that. All I can say is how wrong I was to be scared as staff on Jefferson ward were so won-derful. Nothing was too much trouble for any of them.

'Life can't stop when you are a mum with terminal cancer'

I have always been a huge fan of the late great Freddie Mercury and am not embarrassed to say I cried on the day that he died (everyone is now thinking I have lost the plot and am beginning to ramble. Well, you are, aren't you?). The on-call doctor that night was a slightly darker version of good old Fred and I know, as stupid as it sounds, I think this was why I liked him straight away. Oh, these brain tumours of mine! He was at great pains to discuss everything with me. Every time he received another blood count report he would knock on my door and come in with a lovely smile and say "More good news for you". My white blood cell count wasn't a wonderfully healthy figure but it showed that I wasn't in a dangerous, life-threatening situation. Both my blood pressure and temperature were slightly above normal but, again, nothing much to worry about. So in the end we are still not quite sure if I had a chemo overload or a stomach bug.

I became very sick just a few hours after arriving home, I think due to the medication I was given. This continued for a full two hours but by 7am, although still uncomfortable with my stomach cramps, the worst of two weeks of illness had at last gone.

Last Tuesday, I had my three-weekly drip and saw my consultant Doctor Murray. They were still unsure as to why I have been so unwell; the only way of now finding out was to put me back on my normal dosage of chemo. If, by the weekend, I am in pain again, then we will know the reason why, and my dosage will be decreased by 25%.

If all stays good, then we will know it will have been a long, nasty bug, which is quite likely as my immune system is low. Hopefully, one way or another, the mystery of the pain will be resolved soon.

Now that seems to have passed, I am very miserable with a cold. That is not good, as colds and me do not have an amicable partnership. Knowing my luck, I will have fought cancer for five years (not forgetting, of course, those years when I actually did have cancer but was told that the intrusive lump I was carrying around with me was just a part of me!) and die from a cold as I am not so sure how good my lungs are at present.

I am lucky I haven't had many colds over the years of living with low immunity, but when I do get one it is worse for me than living with cancer as I honestly cannot cope with that sort of illness. I am dosing myself up with lots of remedies, but not taking life as easy as I should. I hope it all doesn't pull me down too far and that I will still be around next week to write a further column. Isn't it so silly to have to worry about a cold?

Wednesday last week was my dreaded day of Francesca leaving our wonderful school, Stoke by Nayland. She cried throughout the day, then came home and stayed under this huge black depressive cloud for

the rest of the evening. She woke up the following day at 11.15am with the words "I'm bored!". Oh the joys of school holidays! As much as she is ready to move on with her school life, I wasn't quite ready for how I felt on the day. My main goal was to get her to this stage of life. The fact that it is coming around far too quickly is very unnerving as it is leading me now to the inevitable and with that, thoughts of dying are now in my mind almost continuously.

As you all know, the school held its charities week in aid of Suffolk Breakthrough Breast Cancer. We had planned a huge raffle but, unfortunately, time seemed to run out. In a way, this was actually quite a good thing as the raffle will now take place in

'Isn't it silly to have to worry about a cold?'

September. During the fundraising we had something very special given to us - a cheque for £532 from Nayland Bowls Club. With this wonderful gesture, readers' donations and all the parents', staff and children's money, the grand total raised was £2,953.68 - and this is without the autumn raffle.

I have spent some time phoning up various shops and stores for gifts. This has shown how generous people can be, but also how certain shops can bluntly refuse even something quite small. Francesca asked me why I wasn't embarrassed to phone up for prizes. I told her a dying mum who wants as much money as possible to go towards researching a hateful disease cannot be proud.

I would just like to finish this week's update with a list of people who are giving or have already given gifts to the school. On behalf of absolutely everyone who will be helped by your understanding and kindness, thank you.

Now for the drum roll please...the winners of "top people of the year" are: Ipswich Town Football Club; Nasser Hussain for his signed cricket shirt; Sudbury Sports; Corncraft, Monks Eleigh; Martin Hogg China, Lavenham; Thorntons, Colchester; The Angel Hotel, Lavenham; Mandy Warner (one of my closest friends); Ski Surf, Colchester; Burton; Etam/Tammy Girl; Virgin Megastore; HMV; Woolworths; Boots; Pizza Town, Sudbury; Cineworld, Freeport; Odeon Cinema, Colchester; All Fired Up, Ipswich; Tesco; Waitrose; Sainsbury's; Rollerworld, Colchester; Colchester Leisureworld; Kingfisher Leisure Centre, Sudbury; JJB Sports; New Look; McDonald's; KFC; Javelin.

Each person I spoke to wished me well. Doesn't it just show that the world can after all, be a nice place?

Rhona x

■ Rhona and Katy would like to thank everyone for their kind donations for the Ladies Driving Challenge. Katy raised £1,367.50, which Archant is matching, taking the total raised to £2,735 for Suffolk Breakthrough Breast Cancer.

August 2, 2004: *Reader's letter touched my heart*

WELL that's it then, my mind has gone missing, most probably swallowed up by those three brain tumours of mine! Hopefully it is only temporary, and it will come back soon.

The reason for knowing it has gone is because I found myself last week trying to teach my dog to speak. Before I realised what I was doing, I was saying: 'Say s-t-r-a-w-b-e-r-r-y, Lily'.

Thankfully, after a few moments, I quickly came to my senses, but, as yet, Lily hasn't said the word!

My cold is still annoying me, but I have managed to get through it very well, in fact, better than I have in 43 years. Usually I am out in the garden in the middle of the night, acting like a banshee, not being able to breathe, but this time I have managed to sleep around the clock and almost feel like facing the world again.

I decided to stay in doors for a week, just in case my body picked up any further nasty bugs. It seems all my previous problems with my stomach have been some sort of a bug, as up to now I haven't had any complications with my chemo dose.

It looks like my old immune system is not playing a fair game with me any more. During one of my early mornings, when I was awake emptying the tissue box, I watched something rather amazing.

Actually, it would not have meant anything to me a few years ago, but now it was something very special and I would imagine, at that time of the morning, I was the only person in the world to see it.

We have a very large and old tree at the bottom of our garden and as I woke up the birds were beginning their dawn chorus. Well, one in particular, because that was the one I watched perched high in the tree, bending its head forward whenever it sang. It stayed there for a good five minutes before it flew away, leaving me knowing that I had woken up to another day of my much-wanted life.

I wonder how many people have ever managed to see such a spectacular sight, when it appears one little bird is singing just for you.

It is now five days since I started to write this and my cold is a lot worse. My doctor has now prescribed antibiotics, as my throat is as sore as it was at the beginning. My eyes are swollen up and my nose has become a constant stream. As for energy, that is now a far distant memory.

I had planned to write much more than this, but I have just received a packed envelope from Katy (Edwards), which includes yet another cheque. Thank you. I will give the cheque to Stoke by Nayland Middle School in September for round two of their fundraising.

The envelope also contained some letters which have made my eyes even more tearful. That *** of a cancer thing, is wrecking many of our lives. Why can't it ever seem to happen to nasty people? Even Kristopher is asking me that now. As a mum, the one thing in life I want and need to happen is that hopefully, one day very soon, research will bring that cure so badly needed.

Anyway, as I was saying, in my package of readers' letters and cards (which I love receiving as they bring me what I need to keep that fight going in me as my health deteriorates) was the following from a reader, who herself has had the worst year imaginable. She took time away from her own sadness and bereavement to write. This will touch everyone, as it did David and myself. So until next week, here is "A letter from Heaven".

To my dearest family, some things I'd like to say

But first of all, to let you know that I arrived OK

I'm writing this from heaven. Here I dwell with God above

Here, there's no more tears of sadness; here is just eternal love

Please do not be unhappy just because I am out of sight

Remember that I am with you every morning, noon and night

That day I had to leave you when my life on earth was through

God picked me up and He said: "I welcome you

It's good to have you back again, you were missed while you were gone

As for your dearest family, they'll be here later on

I need you so badly, you are part of my plan

There is so much that we can do, to help our mortal man

God gave me a list of things, that he wished for me to do

And foremost on the list, was to watch and care for you

And when you lie in bed at night the day's chores put to flight

God and I are closest to you in the middle of the night

When you think of my life on earth, and all those loving years.

Because you are only human, they are bound to bring you tears

But do not be afraid to cry; it does relieve the pain

Remember there would be no flowers,

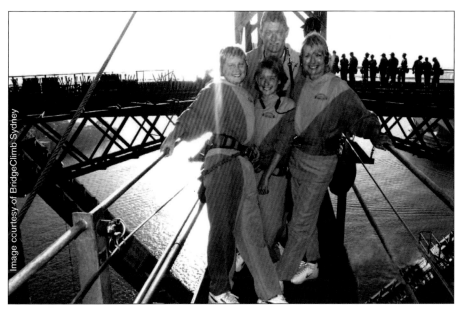

Image courtesy of BridgeClimb Sydney

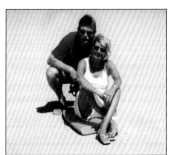

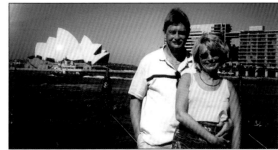

HOLIDAY FUN: Rhona and family enjoy trips to Australia, above, **and Center Parcs,** below

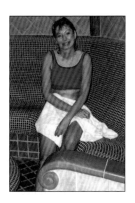

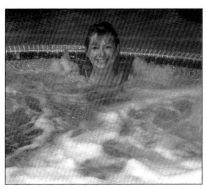

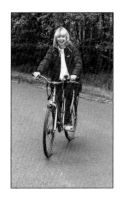

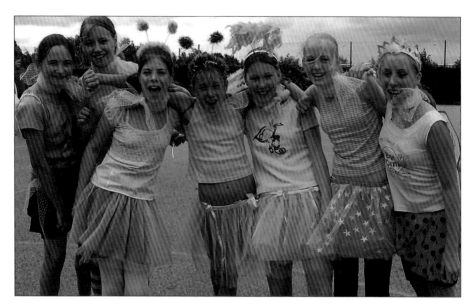

FUNDRAISING FUN: Francesca and some her friends at Stoke by Nayland Middle School during a Suffolk Breakthrough Breast Cancer fundraising activities week

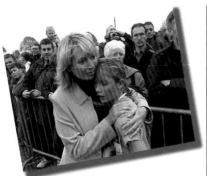

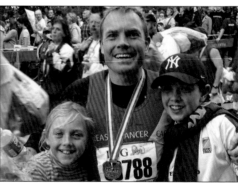

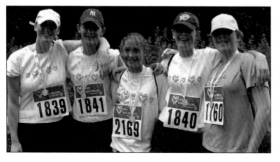

RUNNING FOR THE CAUSE: Paul Excell ran the 2004 New York Marathon for breast cancer cash after being inspired by Rhona. Above, he celebrates with his children James and Jess. Above left, Rhona embraces Francesca after she ran the Race for Life in Norwich and, left, Francesca, centre, with friends who ran the Race for Life with her in Nowton Park, Bury St Edmunds

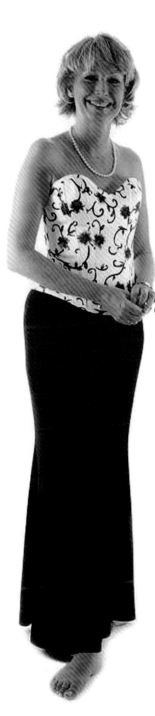

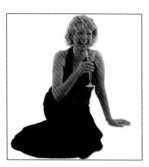

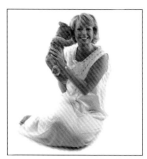

ROLE MODEL: Rhona models specialist clothes by Southwold-based designer Catherine Fuller for women who have had breast surgery. Rhona made such a big impression on Catherine that she also designed a nightwear collection bearing Rhona's name

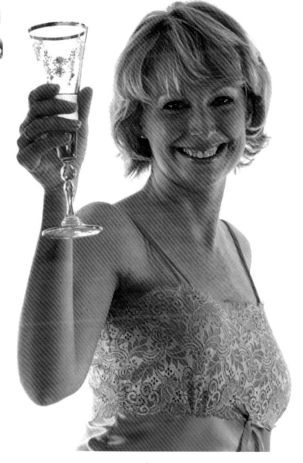

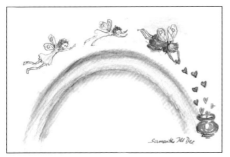

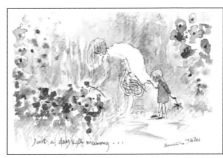

Just a daisy for mummy . . .

ON THE CARDS: Some of the watercolours by Samantha Jill Dee which appear on Rhona's fundraising cards printed by The Panda Group, Haverhill, Suffolk

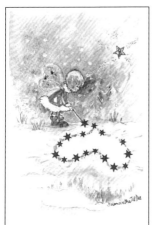

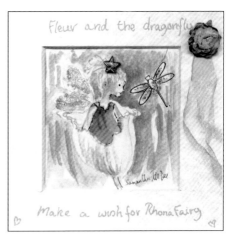

Fleur and the dragonfly

Make a wish for Rhona Fairy

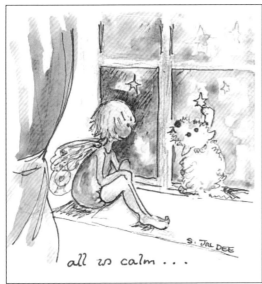

all is calm . . .

S. JILL DEE

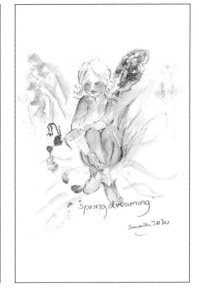

"Spring dreaming"

Samantha Jill Dee

unless there was some rain
I wish that I could tell you all that God has planned
If I were to tell you, you wouldn't under-stand
But one thing is for certain, though my life on earth is o'er
I'm closer to you now, than I ever was before
There are rocky roads ahead of you and many hills to climb
But together we can do it by taking one step at a time
It was always my philosophy and I'd like it for you too
That as you give unto the world, the world will give to you
If you can help someone who is in sorrow or pain
Then you can say to God at night: "My day was not in vain"
And now I am contented that my life was
worthwhile
Knowing as I passed along the way I made somebody smile
So if you meet somebody who is sad and feeling low
Just lend a hand to pick them up, as on your way you go
When you're walking down the street and you've got me on your mind
I'm walking in your footsteps only half a step behind
And when it's time for you to go, from that body to be free
Remember you're not going, you're coming here to me.

After writing this down my cheeks are far from dry, but there are screams of laugher coming from my children downstairs. It's so nice that at times like this they can be so oblivious to real life.

Rhona x

August 16, 2004: *I've been to hell and back*

IT would seem this tough old battleaxe is back - well, forget the "old" part but, through some sort of miracle, I have bounced back.

A week ago I never imagined it would happen. Yet just four days after being told that the most unthinkable thing had happened - a blood clot - I was back to the old me.

So, where do I start? Well, I can only say that I have been to hell and back over the past two weeks. It feels as though I have been on the outside, looking in at someone who was extremely ill and nearing the end of the road on her very last journey.

I have been scared, frightened, tired, emotional, in unbelievable pain and had sickness like I have never known and have often found myself in floods of tears saying: "God, please help me".

My children, David and many of my friends had to watch me decline slowly each day, and there was absolutely nothing they could do about it.

Everyone pleaded with me to eat, but I was in too much pain to even consider a mouthful of food. Instead, all I lived on for a week was water and the odd drink of Lucozade. I was watching my arms and legs turn into those of my mum, as she was weeks before her death. Just walking to the toilet had me bent over with pain and pouring with sweat due to weakness and exhaustion. I wasn't able to sleep as there didn't seem to be a comfortable way of trying to forget the pain.

To top it all, I also had a chest infection. My hope of seeing Francesca start at the upper school was looking very unlikely.

Just when you think things can't get any

worse, they always do. As I was taking yet another tablet, at 8pm on August 5, I felt an unusual pain just by my ribs, on my right side. It got worse and had soon spread under my arm and the whole area surrounding my mastectomy and reconstruction scar.

I didn't say anything to David, as I decided initially that it was all in my mind. As the night progressed, so did the pain. By 3am I was pretty sure I was having a heart attack, so went and kissed each of my children and whispered to them how much I loved them.

I returned to bed and just waited for the end to happen. I decided not to wake David, as I thought it better that he slept as much as possible, as he would need his strength over the next few days. I waited and waited, thinking of how my dad died in just 90 seconds with his heart attack, but no shining lights or even beautiful singing was happening. So I continued to wait.

'I returned to bed and waited for the end to happen'

All that happened was the pain got worse and so did David's snoring. I have always said that when the time comes, I would like my family and closest friends there, with them drinking champagne, laughing and sharing memories. But no, what was I getting? My beloved husband's grunting snorts. What a way to die, eh?

As the hours passed, I went off the idea of having a heart attack (as I would have gone by then). I still knew I had some sort of an infection. My friend Gina took me up to Essex County Hospital, where I had the needle which I don't like, and the word "clot" first entered my life. After the horror of clot, the next word was worse. Heparin - a daily injection into my stomach to thin my blood. For me, that was the very worst thing - needles without wimp cream! To say it was an "ouch" was an understatement.

I was assigned a great (and gentle) district nurse for the next three days, before having my fifth and final injection at my routine hospital appointment on Tuesday. I now have five little black spots on both sides of my tummy. Pretty gorgeous, or what?

A VQ scan was arranged for me on Wednesday. That was a world apart from other scans. A VQ scan means ventilation perfusion, which measures the air and blood flow to the lungs.

The staff at Colchester General Hospital were great and the scan was in no way upsetting. I had to close my mouth around a mouthpiece and have my nose clipped tightly. I then breathed for four minutes, as normally as possible. Not very easy when you still have the remains of a cold and a nose that won't release air.

A series of images are taken before dye has been injected into the system and more images taken. It takes about 40 minutes in all. At 7pm that same evening my doctor from hospital rang me to say: "Have a great holiday." In other words my clot had dispersed and I was fit enough to fly.

So, that brings us back to the beginning. The main point of my diary this week is I have survived again, even though there have been three times over the past three weeks when I felt too weak to continue fighting.

I did it again and all because of the love and help from David, K & F, friends and the many letters and cards I have been sent by readers.

I received another huge package this

morning. It is the best start to anyone's day, knowing you are being thought of and prayed for, but also knowing that I am helping others through this stupid, daft, pathetic, annoying "C" thing.

Many other things are happening over the next couple of weeks but I think if I write any more, no one else will get a look in. So until next Monday, a huge thank you to everyone for all your support when I needed it most...I'm afraid to say I'm still around!! - but feeling just a little proud of myself!

Rhona x

PS: Guess who doesn't need the wimp cream anymore? Me!

August 23, 2004: *Diving into a frenzy of holiday cleaning*

AS I write this, the Damant household is in chaos ... no change there then! We are off to Gatwick tonight and then flying to Sharm el-Sheikh tomorrow morning (Thursday, August 20) for two weeks.

I booked this holiday on the spur of the moment on the first Saturday when I started my cold. David had gone to Tesco, the children were out and I was bored sitting on the sofa surrounded by boxes of tissues, trying to find something interesting to watch on television.

I was failing miserably, when I came across this holiday channel (unlucky for David's credit card!).

By the time he returned (with half of the shopping list missing ... again!), I had convinced myself of what a good idea this was, as I would see Kristopher hopefully gain his PADI diving certificate, which I never thought would be possible.

Even before the shopping was unloaded, I was on that phone with all of David's card details and that was it; a few moments later we were booked to fly off to the Red Sea.

As this was four weeks before I went to "hell and back", I didn't have the slightest idea of what lay in store for me. As it happened, however, the holiday just served to put me under extreme pressure, as I had got everyone all excited about it and it was beginning to look like it was going to have to be cancelled. My energy was non-existent, with my strength not much better, but the most frightening aspect of it all was the possibility of a DVT following my blood clot.

Anyway, as you all know, that is now ancient history and late last week, following my VQ scan, my doctor at the hospital said I was clear to fly.

Still, with less than 24 hours until takeoff, there is still no sign of that usual holiday excitement, as all of us know (and as I have already proved), anything could happen to me at any time.

But, as usual, with my family lack of high emotions doesn't mean calmness so, just like any other year, the house is in madness!

Like all of the rest of the female population, going on holiday always means one thing ... cleaning the house ... which always leads to "words" between David and myself as to why this needs to be done!

This year I promised it would be different, given that I am still very tired, so one of my closest and dearest friends took three days leave from work to help us all get ready. I'm not sure if we could have done it without her, as she kept ordering me around to sort things out!

I don't seem to have any concept of time any longer and can honestly say I am worse than both my children put together. I will get up in a morning and, before I know it, it is almost time for the children to return from school and I won't have a clue to as to what I have managed to spend all my day doing!

As for my memory, well that has become quite a joke for everyone who knows me, as it just doesn't exist any more.

I had my hair cut last Monday and then got a phone call halfway through asking me where was I, as I had also booked myself in for a facial at the same time! Needless to say, my face lost the battle that time!

Steph returned to work today, confident that we were ready for the off, but guess what? I decided to clean the house again, even though it was clean and tidy. I think I will somehow never rid myself of that need to clean before leaving home for two weeks.

Blimey, I have just thought of something - what am I going to do when the time comes for me to leave for good?

I was told during the week by the airline that I needed a letter from my doctor if I wanted to pre-board the aircraft (before everyone else), to say that I was fit enough to fly. Had I known this earlier, I would have asked for one from my hospital doctor, but I didn't want to risk getting in touch and have them decide I actually needed another Heparin injection.

So I asked my own GP if he could write me one. I very much like him and have been his patient for 14 years. He has a very caring and understanding attitude, so I was somewhat taken back when I was told that this letter was to cost me £10!

I have always thought of my surgery as a family practice - it just goes to show that business is the name of the game in the 21st Century.

Insurance, naturally, was going be a huge problem for me, as I was still on treatment. Anyone taking any sort of drug for three months before travel is considered a huge risk. As if it wasn't bad enough me having been on cancer treatment for 14 months, I then go and have a clot! It took me several hours phoning just about everyone to try to find some sort of cover. It seemed the best anyone could offer was a premium of £269 but then an excess of £5,000!

We decided we had no choice but to go with it ... that was, until I found an absolutely brilliant company who seem to deal only with those in a similar situation to myself.

Again we had to pay almost £300, but our excess is just £60, and that covers the whole family, if something were to happen due to my cancer. For anyone who may need cover like this in the future, they are Freedom Insurance Services Ltd, on 0870 774 3760, and are based in Cambridge.

Due to the recent situation with my health, for the first time in five years, I started to get very angry that this could have been allowed to happen to me through what can only be described as negligence.

'Tiredness is my body's way of telling me it needs help'

What is sickening me so much is that a doctor from my area is having to go to the High Court in London and will probably be struck off for having an affair with a patient. Granted, this is not the correct thing to do in life, but he did go on to stay with the person in question.

But the three doctors who had me down as having a hormonal lump, asthma, a 100-day cough (whatever that may be!) and many other mis-diagnoses, are still practising without any question, and are living a lovely life, while I am losing mine.

I have, therefore, asked for the help of one of my friends to look into all of this when I return from holiday. It's now time for me to get answers to my questions so watch this space ... who knows what I will find!

Well, I'd better get moving; I've just got the bath left to clean. .

I intend to chill out and spend most of my time under the shade of an umbrella watching my son go forward into his adulthood - oh, and drink Pimms or the equivalent and read the trashiest novel possible!!!

Rhona x

August 30, 2004: *Am I an old hag, a snake or a fat piggy?*

THE hotel is lovely, food good, the beer nicely chilled, weather (too) hot each day and the mum of one of our reps reads my column, so: "Hi to Matt's mum!"

I am not sure how he and his colleague worked this out but it seems that, after fleeing from our awful summer weather, I have been tracked down to Sharm el-Sheikh.

I really shouldn't be surprised that I have been recognised because when I stop to think about it I am the only person who hasn't changed colour in a week and only tend to poke my nose from under the umbrella about 15 minutes before sunset each evening.

Being in Egypt brings back some lovely memories of how David and I met. We both worked in the Middle East and used to enjoy the heat. The main souks and markets haven't changed much, except that the roads are now made of cobblestones instead of sand.

I can't decide if I am an old hag, a snake or a fat piggy, so I will be all three. On my first trip to Cairo more than 20 years ago, the stallholders shouted after me: "Hey English (despite being Irish), beautiful lady, I show you what I have." But now I am ignored and it is Francesca who gets them all calling after her which begs the question: "Am I jealous that she is beautiful and I am the ignored 'old hag' - the mother." Well of course I am, but I'm also proud that my little girl is turning into a little stunner.

Due to still being haunted by chemotherapy, I am shedding layers of skin on the palms of my hands and soles of my feet (a common side-effect).

In fact, I'm a complete mess as far as my skin is concerned right now as I am just far too hot. Hence, my reference to being a snake. As for the fat piggy part, well that's due to the all-inclusive board we are on - I was brought up never to leave food!

Unfortunately, I have spent 36 hours in bed with what seems to be my three-weekly dose of chemotherapy stomach pains. I thought I could stop this by coming off my drugs for a month but it just goes to show that the chemotherapy is continuing to work in my body.

I did not eat or drink during this time, so put myself into a dehydrated exhaustion, but it was nice the following day, as I had a nice slim middle. Unfortunately, it was soon back to the old, piggy fat me again when those pancakes were served up for breakfast.

AS you know, I decided to come out here in the hope that Kristopher would be able to pass his PADI open diving certificate in what I believe is the most colourful sea in the world. In just one day, I hope he will pass this qualification and make me into a proud old mum again.

He has worked very hard, and is often asleep, fully clothed, by 8pm. To get up each morning at 7am to sit exams in a stuffy classroom before going diving is enough to exhaust anyone just thinking about it. Then there is the fact that all his classmates are at least twice his age. He has told me several times that he is doing it all for me, and I know he is. But I also know it is what he wants and that is the main thing.

So has all this heat fatigue been worth it? You bet it has. To watch my big son on his final three dives on Friday will be one of my proudest moments as a mum. Just being there will be a dream come true as it is yet another achievement I will have shared with my children.

I'm afraid to say that David, Francesca and myself have been very chilled out and lazy during our first week here as K's diving has been the priority. But next week, it will be Brits at their best! We have booked to go to Cairo, quad biking, watching the underwater life from a submarine (I decided this was best the best option for me as there was no exercise needed).

We have also booked to visit St Catherine's Monastery and a cruise for the day. I think, however, I will let the others be the energetic ones, while I chill out near the beer for which I am now famous.

And afterwards? Well, afterwards I will be able to say that's another good family holiday at an end and one which I didn't think I would have. But that's not a problem as I am already planning our next one - just don't tell David.

There are two questions which have been troubling me over the past few days. Why do the British all have brand new white trainers when they go off on holiday (two of my own included) and why, oh why, do other nationalities have to snorkel in the swimming pool each day when they are just five minutes from the sea? Particularly as, in this case, it is one of the world's most beautiful seas? Answers on a postcard to ...

Rhona x

September 6, 2004: *Ready to find another goal to aim for*

IN just two hours we will be returning home from our very adventurous holiday.

I had spent an hour writing my column but the power went down here and all my work disappeared! As time is running out this will be a quick and condensed diary, but when back home I will write more.

The main news is that Kris passed his PADI open diving certificate and went on to pass his advanced qualifications. It will probably mean us re-mortgaging our house but to say I was proud is a huge understatement. In the last two weeks I have watched my son start to mature into adulthood and seeming to need me less and less.

Francesca and I have been inseparable and I now know she is ready to accept what the future holds whether it is close or far away. In just four days I will have reached what at some stage seemed like an unachievable goal - seeing my little girl start at upper school. My health has held up very well for most of the time out here, which means one thing - another great holiday to give us all many happy memories. I have managed to get some colour but, most of all, this holiday has given me back "ME". When we left, I was looking as if I wouldn't pass my next MoT but now I feel great and ready to find another goal to aim for. Next time I will be writing all about our time in Sharm el-Sheikh. Blimey, that sounds as though I'm about to change the world with a huge exclusive - sorry to disappoint you, it will only be the usual from the normally dysfunctional Damant family.

Rhona x

September 13, 2004: *Holiday over, it s down to earth with a bump*

We had a lovely homecoming from our holiday, thanks to some friends. My favourite lilies in a vase ready to bloom, next day's lunch prepared, and all we needed for breakfast.

We hit our much-loved and missed beds at 3am, expecting not to see much of that day but - bing, bong - at 7.30 I was wide awake! I couldn't believe how great I felt, so one of my friends came around and spent the day with me.

Apparently, according to two friends, I had a "tired face" when I left (in other words I looked rough!), but seemingly now looked fantastic. Aren't thousands of freckles covering a face a wondrous thing?! The Sunday morning had me telling David that I was going to start decorating, but as usual in my life the old thunderbolt managed to destroy the good feeling, and by mid-afternoon I was doubled up with stomach cramps again.

'The old thunderbolt managed to destroy the good feeling'

Now, usually I put this down to my chemo, but at the time I wasn't sure if it was that or the good old Egyptian cuisine! But as I write this, on my way home from the Marsden, they are just as bad, if not worse. It's starting to look like my body is rejecting my "wonder drug."

I have had two appointments this week - talk about an abrupt ending to a holiday!

Colchester on Tuesday for my much-needed drip, and London today to see my eye consultant. The news today was good, the tumours behind my right eye haven't changed since January.

I have been given my next appointment for March 10 - it was a weird feeling looking at it, as I'm not sure that I will make that one. This feeling changed to sadness for me when the woman behind was fully discharged, having been clear from her cancer for five years. I would have given anything to have been her, when her husband and children gave her a huge hug and kisses, I sat down and watched them leave a very happy family knowing that all her cancer and treatment was now a closed chapter. They were walking out of that outpatients department to start living a new and wonderful life, and as I could feel the tears, there was that same old voice asking why wasn't it me?

My doctor at Colchester reduced my chemo dosage, but said if the stomach problems continued I would have to come off it - not good news, as the loss of this means that this stupid cancer could start its rampage throughout my system again. Unfortunately, it is day three now and the pains don't seem to want to go, so have I run my course on this one? I hope not, but I don't know. I do have a CT scan in two weeks' time, with a follow-up at the Marsden, so up until some answers are given, it would be nice if this old "bod" of mine could start to behave itself!

I came home to a huge package of cards, letters and CDs from what my daughter now refers to as my "fan club". Fancy me being just like Donny Osmond (guess who joined his fan club in the 70s?) It was so lovely spending Saturday morning with a cup of tea reading all the letters. You always seem to put so much thought into your words of comfort and encouragement. I hope you all know how much this means to me - thank you.

Well, the memories of Egypt now and where do I start? It was a holiday full of highs, with the only low that it has given David a new balance on his credit card - again!

It has given me a lot of reassurance that we have started to set K up for his gap year, which he has already decided he is having - and in Australia, if you please! As long as he joins a sub-aqua club here and continues with his dive training, by the time he goes on his travels he will be able to give fruit-picking a miss to top up his funds, instead being able to dive for a living. What a life that would be, eh?

As I have said, I was so proud of him, but could have easily throttled him when he said: "Well, personally, I prefer the Great Barrier Reef to dive in."

Cairo was fascinating to the rest of the family, but I found myself thinking back 16 years ago on my last visit there (when I was cabin crew) when I rode all around the pyramids then down to the Sphinx on a camel. Now air-conditioned coaches have taken the place of the uncomfortable camel, and buildings like the KFC are starting to surround what was once a desert. Lunch was on the Nile, but then afterwards I had someone ask me if I was pregnant? The thing was she was about three times the size of me!!

Three of us spent a day on a sun-seekers cruise, which initially I was slightly wary about, as often these sort of things are very touristy.

But how wrong I was. It turned into day I will never forget. Miles away from the coastline in the most turquoise of water, with classical music playing, along swam five wild dolphins. The sight was so amazing.

But so were the men on the boat, as they pushed aside the smaller of the females so that they could have a better view. Whatever happened to manners?

The four of us became rebels for a few hours as we went out quad biking to watch the sunset deep into the desert. I think we all looked like little Lego people, with our crash helmets on, but we didn't care as the excitement of it all was really something else. We missed the sunset, of course, but we ended up having tea with the Bedouins. It was totally an eye-opener, and at first I felt huge sorrow for the little children, as they had so little, and were so grateful when we bought some little handmade bracelets for a few pence.

But as we left I thought about how happy they all were - they didn't have the pressures that we all tend to put ourselves under, their smiles were heart-warming, and just watching them as we rode away I came to the conclusion that, unlike us, they probably didn't have a worry in the world!

I could continue to write pages about our hols, but I would bore you all to sleep, so I am just going to finish on a funny note.

I will never know if this was meant as a compliment, chances are it wasn't, but I will always think and smile about it. When you go into the souk, the traders shout at you - "hey English ... you want Asda price ... buy one get one free", always followed by "lovely jubbly". As you can imagine it gets quite irritating after a while.

On our last night there, Francesca and I went out girlie shopping with a lady who we had become quite friendly with. We hadn't had anything to drink so what happened next just goes to show how alcohol is not needed to make a fool of oneself.

As soon as we arrived we attracted all of their daft sayings, so when one came after us shouting: "You, English" we turned round and said: "We know what you're going to say." With which he replied: "No...you..the dogs b*****ks!"

When I did finally walk away with tears of laughter running down both cheeks, I immediately bumped into what had to be the biggest painting in Egypt, knocked it down, stand and all, that in turn made the next one fall, and so the three of us left, leaving the local people asking each other what on earth had that been all about?

OK sleepy-heads, you can wake up now!

My big goal was of course achieved last Monday, with Francesca starting at the upper school.

All went smoothly, and it was like any other first day of term, but for me the feelings were more than just: "Yes, I've got my space back!"

Rhona x

September 27, 2004: *New strength from an unexpected visitor*

IT is good to be writing that this very old, worn rubber ball has regained some of its bounce, and is around for that little bit longer. Actually, maybe I am the dog's "wotsits" after all!

A week ago, it certainly looked and very much felt that I had reached the final road and, as far as I was concerned, I wasn't going to walk off it this time. To be honest, I was feeling so weak, with lack of food and fluid, experiencing pain which I am sure will not be as bad as that, even at the end, I could for the first time in five years see how easy it is to give up.

And that was what it seemed I was then starting to do. Due to my last horrific memory from the Marsden, when I was a patient in February, I fought going back into hospital when that's where I should have been.

My bed, then, was next to a dying woman, who I could watch throughout the night, bringing back all the painful reminders of when my mum died.

Just watching her son and daughter cry, sleeping across her for minutes at a time, not leaving her side, just in case the time came and they weren't there to hold her hand, quite frankly scared me from ever wanting to go in for overnight treatment again.

But, how stupid was I? Not only did I endure a week that can only be described as the worst time yet, I dehydrated myself so much that when I finally knew the time had come to give in, I ended up having 106 hours of continuous fluids!

That, however, wasn't the only stupid thing. I didn't think for one minute of how the staff (at Colchester) would be the complete opposite of those in London!

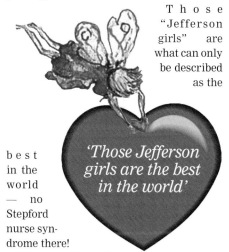

Those "Jefferson girls" are what can only be described as the best in the world — no Stepford nurse syndrome there!

'Those Jefferson girls are the best in the world'

They are there for every emotion and the "pampering" is now being missed by yours truly!

But do you know what the difference is from any other ward of which I have been a guest? They choose to be there, and for them, it isn't just a part of their training which they have to do.

This palliative ward is where they all

shine through, with hands willing to be squeezed until they are broken when that needle is put in, a cup of tea in the night when the going seems to be tougher than ever and, of course, the gentleness of just knowing that they are there for "us", the patients.

What more is there to say? Essex Rivers staff, I will, when the time comes, grant you all dustings of my fairy powder!

As usual with me, I can't be happy with just having major dehydration so, to add a little more spice to my life, on the Saturday night, just after David and the children went home, my temperature rose and my body decided to have a party with an infection!

A lovely young doctor came to take a "jam jar" full of blood from me and then I had even more fluids fed into my arm with antibiotics. The funniest thing was that Donny Osmond was on television and the nurse who ended up having the obligatory broken fingers, which I am now known for, was the same age as me.

We knew all the words of *Puppy Love*, as we had both bought it in our teens. The saddest thing of all was this young doc hadn't a clue who this old man on TV was, as he had been born in 1979!

When I found out he had been born in Australia, the idea did cross my mind: aha, a passport to Oz, should I ask him to marry me? (Forgetting David, of course!)

But when I worked out how old he was, the realisation hit me that he could be my son! So come back David, I really didn't mean it!!

On this night of infection, the strangest thing that has, or probably will ever, happen to me occurred. Before I tell you, I will just say that I am one of the world's biggest sceptics, and when I read articles of how people had near-death experiences I normally dismiss it as wanting £500 for the best story of the week in that particular paper!

But I'm not about to sell my story to the *News of the World*.

Just after all the "excitement (?)" of my latest health scare ended, I was lying on my bed, just thinking, with my eyes closed. I was too awake to go to sleep, so resting was just nice. I then felt someone sitting beside me, but when I looked, no one was there, and I knew a nurse hadn't come into my room.

I closed my eyes again, to feel that warmth of someone who is sitting close to you and then there he was: my lovely dad. When I say he was there, I couldn't see him, but he was there with me. When I closed my eyes I saw him in a cardigan, which I bought him with my first ever pay packet. He hadn't aged, he was just how I remembered him.

The comfort of my dad being with his little "girlie" again was the most gorgeous feeling I have ever experienced.

I thought he had come to take me with him, and I was ready to go, just happy knowing that he would take my hand and bring me back to where I belonged with him and my mum.

Knowing that he was there gave me the most wonderful sleep and the best one I have had for years. I woke at 5am, and he had gone, without me.

I knew then that he had been there to get me through yet another night and to give me back my strength to carry on fighting and watch both my little girl and boy grow up that little bit more.

Now, Francesca's entrance into adulthood, with her starting upper school. It was, 15 months ago, my main, but most likely unachievable goal. I have found out now that few expected me to do it (including myself) but on Monday, September 6, I was there to wave off her, Kristopher and Irene (my children's life-long friend who lives opposite) on what went on to feel just like every other first day of term! Nothing different happened, champagne corks didn't appear to go off in my tummy, and I certainly didn't drape myself in bunting, telling the world that I had done it.

It was just another ordinary day!

I did, however, feel apprehensive throughout the day, wanting them both to come home and tell me all. I didn't go out, but seemed to constantly keep an eye on the clock until 4pm.

Then the back door opened, silence left the house, bags were dropped, followed by shoes here and there, and both disappeared into their bedrooms with just a "Hi mum". End of story!!

Unfortunately, Francesca, for the first time in her life, dislikes the school and also, for the first time ever, she has been given ridiculous detentions.

She arrived from Stoke (Middle) with just four other girls, but she was the segregated one and has had to find her bearings at a huge school without the help of girls she knew.

She seems to have gone from a prize pupil to one that will very soon lose all interest in her neatness and desire to work to please the teacher as, it seems, for certain subjects there, she is at fault for just about everything. I have already spoken to the school, but as yet I have not seen any change.

On Saturday, when she spent the day at hospital with me, she worked throughout the day on schoolwork, only to have a comment written on a piece of work: "Did she actually spend at least half an hour on her work?" Well, Mr or Mrs Maths Teacher, she spent one-and-a-half-hours on her work, and I was there watching it.

I have come to the conclusion that the pupils who don't want to learn seem to be the pupils the teachers bow to. But those like my daughter, who has worked throughout her school life and who, on occasions, I have found at 2am working on a subject, are the ones who some teachers tend to have the inclination to upset.

My child was never going to be a Cambridge graduate, but the way her schooling is going, she will be lucky to leave school at 16 with any confidence at all.

Next week will be my first anniversary of "diary writing". Who would have thought that, one year on, I would be fatter than ever but, more importantly, still here!

Rhona x

October 4, 2004: *Still determined to live and love life*

SO, here it is, the last year's memories of the highs and lows of living with cancer! I never thought when I started my diary 12 months ago that I would be sitting writing this now.

To even plan our holiday to Australia was a big enough goal. But to get through four seasons, to live to what seemed like the unreachable target of waving my daughter off to upper school, seemed, with my prognosis of terminal cancer in just about every part of my body, unmanageable. But here I am, still living the lives of two people; one with healthy good days and the other of a cancer-ridden, very tired and at times scared woman.

Before I start my ramblings there have been a few happenings last week I would like to tell you about.

Last Monday, I received a lovely letter from a reader containing a cheque for £420, raised by residents of Badwell Ash, after a village fun day.

They have sent it to me to send to Suffolk Breakthrough Breast Cancer. It arrived out of the blue, so I was very surprised and, once again, could not believe it was by reading my column that it was agreed to send this wonderful amount of money to Suffolk's own research branch.

Thank you all so much.

I have been asked many times why I have chosen this particular charity. I suppose it has been for sort of selfish reasons. As you know, I am not Suffolk born and bred, but my children are. In all likelihood they will, in time, leave their roots and look for pastures new, but when it comes to it, your home will always be home. Although it has never been proved that I am a carrier of a cancer gene, it is very likely I am, which will then go further down generations.

Should this nightmare ever decide to appear in our family again, then my children will always know that, through me, the people of Suffolk donated generously to help find what may be one day be a cure for this type of cancer.

When I started writing my column, a reader sent me a copy of Lee Ann Womack's CD, with her favourite track being *I Hope You Dance*. The words were so meaningful. Now, the strange thing is, when we started talking about putting the diaries into print, I was asked who, if it was possible, I would like to have write the foreword. Being a good Irish girl (?) I immediately said Ronan Keating. Well I would, wouldn't I, him being a good Irish boy!

Actually, joking aside, Ronan seemed to be a good choice as he too has suffered by losing a much-loved mum at an early age, due to cancer.

He went on to promote major fundraising in Ireland and is taking a huge part in the awareness month during October. He has also released *I Hope You Dance* and is donating proceeds to charity.

He is a bit of alright and by being young and lovely I would like to think this would get through to the younger age group that breast cancer does not just affect middle-aged women. So, come out Ronan from wherever you are and help me sort out my book, please!

I had a CT scan last Friday at Colchester. I am very used to tests like this now so wasn't unduly worried about it, but I think the fact that it was an enhanced scan of my stomach and surrounding areas made it different. I had to drink one-and-a-half pints of iodine every seven minutes, one-and-a-half hours before the scan (which was new to me) but when the dye was injected I had a very hot feeling run throughout me, which actually made me feel quite sick.

I hope to have the results by the middle of the week as I have an appointment at the Marsden on Wednesday, to see Professor Smith about future treatment. I am not sure what, if any, chemo will be available to me, as I adamantly refuse to lose my hair this time around. I want a quality of life now. If I was offered an extra year of good health, then I could be persuaded, but at this stage the odds would be stacked against that!

If there is to be another drug then I expect it would be given intravenously as I think I have had the only oral chemo drug available. That's all the news up to date. What of the past 12 months?

It is difficult to know where to start, as very little has changed really in the past year. I have managed to sleep through a great deal of it, so it isn't really 12 months, but probably about six. We as a family have spent much more time together, as time is precious now and we need to try to fulfil what dreams we have before time runs out.

There have been a few doubtful times, when it was beginning to look as if time was being called on me. I have to live all our futures and as many goals, events and challenges as quickly as I can, but by doing this I am also wishing what is left of my life away.

In a way, I am forcing my children to grow up more quickly than they should, but at the same time it is a must that I see them do whatever is possible.

Kristopher is now taller than me; although this makes me feel old, I also love it, as I feel he will be capable of looking after his "little" mum when the time comes. They have both started to mature. Granted both of them have times when I feel as if they are driving me insane, but that is no different from other parents of the lovely, grunting teenager. They get away with much

more than they should, but if I do change into my banshee mode, then I spend the next few hours feeling so much guilt it upsets me more than them.

Tiredness is a more frequent visitor now. I smile when I remember the times when I used to think I was tired. How wrong I was. Weariness is a huge part of the illness.

The past year has also brought the loss of some people who I thought of as friends.

Unfortunately, when the terminal diagnosis came, some people went, for reasons known only to them. I cannot waste energy on trying to make people stay there for me when they feel they can't. My circle of friends now are those who are genuine friends and they will always remain there for me, on the days when I feel as if I can't continue with this daft old life of mine.

With writing the column came the chance

'Weariness is a huge part of the illness'

of working on a documentary about living with cancer for Anglia Television. One of the great memories of the past year has been our visit to the studios in Norwich.

Many hours of recordings and retakes have taken place over the months, with the funniest being when Tony and Natalie spent the day at the Marsden with me. I had, among other treatments that day, an eye appointment. What Tony didn't realise was that each drop squeezed into my eye really does sting and leaves me as blind as a bat! One drop is all that is needed, but on this day, with the camera rolling, further drops were being put in so that the recording would be just perfect!

Tony would say "could we just do that again?", and my great eye consultant would say "of course, shall we have another drop then?" Meantime, I was in excruciating pain. Poor old Tone had no idea of what was happening, so I think he has felt guilty ever since, but don't worry, I will still send the nice fairy dust your way.

We haven't reached the end of this snapshot of my dysfunctional family. As I have said, it can continue throughout my short-term life. It's unlikely, therefore, that I will get to see the ending, but I hope it will give an insight of how to live as full a life as possible with the "Big C".

Back in November, I worked with a company who design gorgeous evening and nightwear for women in my situation. With my silicone and the glamour of what will soon be my own collection of specially designed nightwear by Catherine Fuller, I expect I will be asked to take over from Jordan in the next programme of *Celebrity* in the jungle!

My love of fairies, and lavender being my favourite colour, has given Catherine the difficult task of making a "Rhona fairy", which I hope will be sold with my book - I have ideas of tying them together with fairy dust ribbon; proceeds to a cancer charity. I also would like to distribute this package to various cancer/palliative care wards. It has been a very good year for me. OK, there have been a few lows, as in heart operations, lungs collapsing, clots, dehydration... you know, all those silly things that come hand-in-hand with cancer, but I have lived and loved life.

I will never see those important milestones all mums should be allowed to see - children passing exams, learning to drive, weddings and grandchildren. But I know, throughout the past six years since my dad died, he has been there for me. Many times I find myself saying 'thanks dad' or 'thank you dad for not letting something happen'. So I hope that from another life, when the time comes, I will be there to guide my children and for them to know I will always be close by. I don't have a full lifetime ahead of me, but what I am allowed to have I will enjoy, love, but most of all steer my children in the right direction of life.

Someone has to, and that right now is still my job. So on that note, here's to the next year (I hope!).

Rhona x

October 11, 2004: *I hope to see another spring*

I HAVE felt very tired all week and I am wondering if this is how life will be from now on. I manage to get through days by going to bed by 8pm and crossing off the following one, knowing it will be a sleep day!

I think David will be relieved, knowing that constant lunches are a past memory. A close friend has always reminded me of "standards" - make-up etc - but even that is starting to slip. I would prefer to spend that extra five minutes in bed. Oh well David, that's another saving. You'll be able to buy me a garden hot tub soon and I can spend my days soothing away my pains. You see, from what I have heard, it is good for medical conditions (hint, hint Mr D!).

Even though Francesca has left our lovely Stoke by Nayland Middle School, we, as a family, hope to keep in touch. Last Saturday, we visited one of the teachers and had a great day. I had my first ever vegetarian meal, which is a way of life I am just starting on - more about that next week.

You will probably remember how, at the end of last term, many shops and clubs donated goodies to a school raffle for Suffolk Breakthrough. Well, the raffle has been held. As yet I am not sure of the amount raised - news to follow. I had to go back to the Marsden last week, but more heart-breaking was a programme on Caron Keating.

Her death brought home to me how ill I am and, like her, I will leave two children with just memories of a mum. I taped it so I could watch and cry on my own. There were many similarties, which meant I went on to watch it several times, each with tears worse than before.

J ust three days before, I had a conversation with a friend about how thin my legs were becoming. In a way, they reminded me horribly of my mum's in her last couple of months. The one thing that did disturb me was just how thin Caron's legs were. Her cancer had spread to her spine, but with me that is only one of the areas of my body with secondaries, so I have been thinking, 'what hope do I have?'

I don't have the funds they had to try alternative treatments abroad but despite that, she lost her fight.

Wednesday brought the results of my recent CT scan. The spread of cancer presently is under control, with the word "remission" used. To many, this word means "gone". The meaning in Marsden terms is very different. No big celebrations, simply an acceptance that at least it hasn't gone into any new areas. I was given three treatment options: to go back onto the same chemo, at a very low dose, building up as my body allows; secondly if tests prove my ovaries have completely closed down, I could have a hormonal drug, not as powerful as chemo. And the last choice: nothing. The third choice was a non-starter, it is still uncertain whether I could have the middle one, so that left chemo. So next Tuesday - here we go again!

I know at some stage the chemo will stop working, but while it does, I will continue to "do drugs"!

This day was also the one I knew I had to push for a prognosis, which tied my stomach up several times, but after over five years of official diagnosis, the time has come to plan. Prof Smith was very honest and said I will know when it starts to happen. This again haunts me.

About a month before she died, my mum told my dad she knew what was happening as she had seen it before when her niece died of leukaemia. I was then told that my death was unlikely to be a quick one, which I was slightly confused about as I had always thought it would be, due to the likelihood of my lungs or liver giving up. But it would seem not. I was told I would see Christmas (which I never thought I wouldn't and have already arranged a mulled wine party) but to set another goal for six months' time.

Now that causes a problem, as it will be a month from Kristopher's birthday and then two weeks later it is Francesca's. That goal will have to be in eight months! Prof Smith smiled, saying what about a year's goal, but we both agreed that even for me, that was too optimistic.

So that sums up my future - do as much sooner rather than later as it doesn't look too good after the spring.

It's my favourite season so I will be happy if I can see the daffodils just once more. It should also mean that I will see K through to 15 and F having chosen her GCSE options. I never thought I would be allowed to watch my children grow up as long as this, so really I am the lucky one.

Life might have been cruel, but at least they are quite independent young people and although I will be missing their future lives, I know I was their mum during their most important years.

And now I need to go because those silly old tears are arriving again. It hasn't been the best of weeks.

Rhona x

'I'll be happy if I can see the daffodils just once more'

October 18, 2004: *Have pride in your generosity*

THANKFULLY, no tissues this week! Apart from the usual tiredness, all is well on the old health front.

The best news of the week is that Stoke by Nayland Middle School raised the outstanding amount of £1,100 for Suffolk Breakthrough Breast Cancer last week. A huge thank you must go to everyone who made this all possible (again!). Those who donated the prizes, the parents and friends who bought the tickets, and the teachers and staff who gave so much time (and money) to our now very well known local charity. Many cheques have been sent to me over the last few months, which I have now sent on to future research sources - I hope everyone who has joined our fund-raising over the past months feels very proud of themselves, as it is your generosity that means the future for many could look healthier. Now, I must start to plan my next project, my book.

I received two beautiful presents through the post during the week. I used to own a shop in Lavenham (and, yes, to the reader who wrote to me ages ago asking me if I was the "lady" who used to run the flower shop, it is me. But I'm not too sure about the "lady" bit, as I do have my moments!) and became very friendly with many of my customers.

Obviously, as the years have gone by since giving up the shop due to my health, I have lost contact with most of them. So it was very unexpected when two of the prettiest watercolours I have ever seen popped through my door.

Many hours of careful and detailed work created cards especially for me. Jill and Chris, who I met about six years ago, remembered me and my story of how Francesca couldn't understand when she

'We are meeting up to go fairy shopping as we both love them'

was very small why I had given her such an awful name when she could have been called "Twinkle!"

So my painting of the "Twinkle fairy", complete with Rhona's fairy dust, came into my life last Saturday, followed by the "Fleur fairy" on Monday.

It was lovely to make contact again and we are meeting up to go fairy shopping as we both love them so much.

I have asked for Jill's permission have the paintings printed in the book, as not many people have ever had the privilege of having their own special fairy painted just for them.

I went to Colchester for a bone-drip this week, to find out from Dr Murray that I do, in fact, have further options open to me with the chemo route. (I was told at the Marsden the only option was Capecitobine, which made me so ill, again).

It's becoming a nightmare wondering what and who to believe in this cancer world. I have now returned to the drugs, but am taking a very low dose, which probably will not be enough to do much, but Dr M and myself hope that I won't be a guest of the county hospital during this three-week cycle.

When I was there, Chris, the maestro of veins, told me about a new scanner which they hope to buy. It is ultrasound to detect veins on people like myself. What a genius invention this is - but also a costly one at £10,000.

Aahh, a new fund-raising thought! All this goes to show that improvements are being made for us, the "C" people.

I mentioned last week the veggie diet - or actually the lack of it at present! I've not been too good up till now. When I was in hospital last month, GMTV featured a herbal drug from India called Carctol. Although it is mainly associated with pancreatic cancer, there have been rumours of it also helping those like me with secondary breast cancer. I'm not mad enough as yet to think of this as my cure, but often wonder when I read about these so-called miracle drugs, if they do actually work. I know it is only a handful of people they will work for, and for hundreds of others, they don't.

This one, to me, seemed to have that something different about it. As it apparently cost £100 a month, it was accessible enough to have a go. It is also a drug which will, if it works, show results in two months, so again I thought this sounded worth trying.

I contacted the given number to find out that it is only prescribed by 10 doctors in the UK, who also just happen to be from Harley Street.

Yes, you know what is coming next. This £100-a-month drug then becomes a £1,000+ drug, so not at all accessible to ordinary people like myself.

David joked that I should contact GMTV to tell them what I thought about this "carrot", which to his embarrassment, I did!

I spoke to a very irate producer who thought it was perfectly OK to promote this, even though it had hidden costs. In the end we agreed to disagree with their policy.

It is fine to give people diets etc, but to get people excited over what could be that miracle cure for them, only to find it is all too expensive to have, is just not on. Very few people can afford Harley Street costs of a £450 blood test here and a £175 telephone consultation there.

After calming down, I found this little blue drug on the internet at a cost of £120 for a two-month high-dosage supply and it has been shipped directly to me from India. It has to be taken alongside a very strict vegetarian and non-acid diet, as cancer cells live on acid.

This means that most of my favourite comfort foods have to go. I have managed to cut down on many of the forbidden fruits and other goodies, but as yet haven't started on the drug.

I talked it over with Dr M and we agreed that I should start it next month, as we wouldn't be sure if there are any complications with my health over the next few weeks. I will keep you all informed.

Last week saw another birthday for David, whose wife still gives him very stupid cards and pressies.

A year ago, I didn't know what to write on what I thought would be his last card from me. This year I couldn't really do the romantic thing, so I bought him, among other things, a ceramic, rather unpleasant woman which said "she came - she criticised - she went".

So David now has a lasting reminder by his side of the bed of how his wife entered his life, criticised his DIY skills for 20 years, and then she left for a fairy life!

The only thing was that when I explained this to him, I suddenly didn't see the funny side of it any more and almost had to go off to find that box of tissues again. But by then he was opening his boxers which had the same wonderful sentiments on them.

Poor old David!

Rhona x

October 24, 2004: *So tired, even lunch is cancelled*

BEFORE the update from me, I just need to tell you all something very wonderful that happened to me last week but, as usual with my brain, I forgot to mention it!

During my last visit to hospital - wait for it - some lovely person thought I was in my early 30s. Is that a confidence booster, or what? Despite having over a decade removed from my face of horrors, it hasn't made the rest of me feel so much younger.

I am afraid this week won't be my normal epic as, presently, I feel like I have reached the winter in my life and the forecast looks quite bleak over the next few days - well, I hope that's all it will last for!

I have been so tired I have cancelled seeing all my friends this week which has meant missing out on quite a few lunches (oh well, I suppose all of this saving is going to a good cause. No, not David's wallet, but my hot tub!).

I always get up with the children in the morning and get their breakfast ready but one day I couldn't even manage that and ended up waking properly at 3pm!

Pains in my legs also have become more frequent and, having spent most of the last week in bed, I know I will be a prime candidate for bed sores. I can remember my mum having them and the horribleness that went with them, especially the shrill of her scream when my dad used to try to turn her in the bed.

The pain actually wakes me up if I have been lying in the same position too long and then, when I turn, I can guarantee the same pain will repeat itself with that leg.

Walking up and getting down stairs has started to become a struggle and has also started me wheezing again. This is something that has been gradually getting worse over the past few weeks but, when I mentioned it to the Marsden on my last visit, they listened to my chest and said it sounded clear, just like it did for four months before my terminal diagnosis of secondary cancer in my lungs.

I have had a visit from my Macmillan nurse this week and she has advised me to speak to my consultant on my next trip to Essex County, which might mean a chest X-ray, just to make sure problems are not arising again.

I have my lovely friend Sue, who unfortunately has multiple sclerosis, so we can console each other about the tiredness, as she can truly understand the extent of it.

Unless you are actually in this position, it is very difficult for people to fully comprehend. We were both talking about how just washing our hair now takes up a full day's supply of our energy.

The sad thing is, I love going to sleep just as much as I love going out for lunch. Now isn't that a sorry state of affairs!

My very close friend Mandy works at The Angel Hotel and Restaurant in Lavenham, which is on my list of favourite lunching spots. She has asked the owners if they can have a "wear it pink" day in aid of breast cancer care this Friday. Each member of staff then donates £2 with, no doubt, many other donations coming from customers.

Mandy's daughter, Coral, and son, Sam, are also joining in with the pink theme at their places of work and will most likely persuade their friends to do the same!

From what I have heard, even the men at The Angel are taking part. Good on them, is all I can say. Mind you, I have heard that it has been known for people who don't wear the designated colour to be fined £3. Knowing my friend as well as I do, a word of warning - just think, you just might find Mandy behind you with her pink bucket!

Thanks must go to The Angel for taking part in a cause so close to many hearts.

I had a very slight insight last week into how David must feel when I have surgery, as my little dog Lily went in to be spayed. I couldn't even take her to the vet's myself and gave the dreadful job to my friend Mary. I spent all day in a cloud of stress and phoned up as soon as I could to find out how she was. I was so out of control, not being able to do anything. Lily has become my little baby. I know, daft isn't it, but I love her so much. She is totally my little companion and is always by my side.

Just sitting around all day, watching the

clock and feeling scared that anything could happen to her, put me where David has been on occasions with me. He, though, had to be brave for me and try not to show huge amounts of emotion, to stop me from falling apart. Of course, with Lily I didn't have to go through this.

I don't think I have ever before really sat down and thought about just how it all must have affected David.

To have walked alongside my hospital bed, holding my hand and then giving me that final kiss, not knowing what the end result would be, must have been absolute hell.

Apart from the last op when he wasn't allowed to see me afterwards, as I was in intensive care, he has always been there for me as soon as I came round, but not once

have I ever thought what he must have been feeling until I lived all of this out last week.

Thankfully, my Lily is fine but she has become even more spoilt than she was before, and now sits at the top of the stairs every morning waiting to be carried down.

I am having a problem with my words today, I am typing all the wrong things, so I hope the spell-check is working well.

But it's not been just today that it has been like this. I have had trouble with speaking all week. Sometimes I have had to have quite a few attempts trying to make my sentences understandable - maybe I'm just tired.

Oh, well, I'll go back for my peaceful little rest!

Rhona x

November 1, 2004: *School break means I get much busier*

HAVING seen little else but my four bedroom walls over the past couple of weeks, I decided it was time to remove myself from my lovely warm slumber.

Thankfully, this coincided with half term, as being constantly tired doesn't mean a thing when two teenage children need my taxi several times a day.

Granted, I have pushed myself much more than I should have, meaning I will pay highly for it in the week, but during school holidays my life is too short to give in to sleep when K & F want life to be as normal as possible.

Last Monday, they had both arranged days with their friends, which gave me time for lunch!

Actually, I have been out three times to eat, one being with Francesca. It would seem Kristopher prefers a sandwich with his best mate, Jonno, rather than being seen out with his old dear mum!

Oops, it looks like I've become that embarrassing mother I have always wanted to be. However, unlike my mum used to do when I was out with her, I don't sing along with songs in shops; well, not yet anyway!

One lunch was with Jill and Chris, who I have talked about recently, Jill being the artist of the beautiful "Twinkle fairy" you see on these pages. Since rekindling our friendship, I now have a wonderful selection of watercolours and drawings, which Francesca and I adore.

Three of her masterpieces are very Christmassy, so I am looking into having them printed and made into Christmas cards, with all the proceeds going to cancer causes. Obviously time is marching very quickly towards 2004's festive season so, if we can make it happen, it has to be in the next few weeks. I should know whether it's possible by the time that I write next week's diary- but wouldn't it be so exciting if it all went ahead?

Spending money comes quite naturally to my daughter and me so where else should we go but our old favourite, the Corncraft complex?

I ate there with Jill and Chris on Monday and then F and I went back on Tuesday with my friend Sue and her daughter Melanie. We are now trying to make a point of taking the girls who are similar in age out once every school holiday, as they have one very major thing in common: their mums!

As I have mentioned before, Sue and I have our extreme tiredness moments which we console each other about, but from time to time our scatty moments too, so it is nice for our daughters to compare notes!

Lunch number three was made by my great neighbour, Paula, who made all my favourites! I love my soup, and during times of great fatigue this is about all I can manage to eat, so I am very lucky as Paula is always there to make me several days' supply of my main diet.

What would I do without all my friends?

The pains in my legs have become more powerful over the past week and are waking me up a lot more than they used to.

Whereas I used to be able to sleep for long periods on each side, I am now only managing about an hour before I need to move myself, slowly, onto the other side again.

Until I had my mastectomy almost five years ago, I used to always sleep on my tummy but, with a silicone implant as part of reconstruction, this now makes it impossible as it just doesn't flatten and has the right-hand side of me reaching for the stars!

It took quite a long time to get used to side sleeping, so it's annoying to say that the pain is getting in the way of a good night's sleep.

It is quite difficult to describe how the pain feels, as it is nothing I have ever experienced before. The only way is to try to think of being a person without skin, with bones feeling brittle and thin. During sleep it feels as if all of the body's weight is lying on just that bone - it is not a sharp pain, but a heavy one, as if someone had just gone mad with a sledgehammer.

When I move it doesn't go away immediately; at night it seems to take forever to go, but when it finally does, I know in a short time that the hammer will have hit the other side.

I just wish that it would go away and leave me alone, but somehow I know it is here to stay.

October breast care awareness month has now finished for another year. Apart from the article which was printed in the EADT at the beginning of the month, I also did an interview for Radio Suffolk with Lesley Dolphin, which was exciting for me and, for those who don't read this column, enlightening about the everyday life of someone with cancer.

'What would I do without all my friends?'

I appeared in two articles for magazines after being asked by Breakthrough Breast Cancer.

One was for *Prima*, which included David talking about how cancer affects our life (I seemed to be the only one with terminal cancer, the other two couples had gone back to getting their lives as much together as possible).

The other, for *Woman*, was how to speak to a child about a parent being seriously ill. A counsellor then writes how she would do it, so I was pleased when I seemed to get it right. Even though my children were quite young at the time, I was always truthful with them. Changes were going to happen in our daily life and, of course, still do, so it is best that they know exactly from either David or myself the truth, rather than their minds going berserk with the unknown.

I did ask also for outside help from the hospice, which some people have frowned upon, but I know for us this was the best approach as feelings can often be released to someone who is not a family member or friend.

I would be a fool to think that everything is wonderful for my children, of course it's not, but I know they can ask me absolutely anything and I will answer them truthfully.

On the whole it's been a good week. Next week I am back to hospital for my beloved bone-drip, and hopefully an idea as to why my cough has reappeared again.

I hope I will have lots of news about the cards and how both The Angel in Lavenham and Corncraft got on with their "wear it pink" days.

I'm off to have a look at the remaining autumn leaves. I love the colours and the thought that I have been allowed to watch this for another year.

Rhona x

November 8, 2004: *Getting the giggles, by royal appointment*

IT'S been an all-coughing and all-giggling week! My cough has advanced enough for my hospital consultant to prescribe either methadone or liquid morphine to help people around me enjoy a quieter life.

Both I have tried before and both I dislike. My chosen route this time is the morphine as it has been prescribed at quite a low dose.

As yet I haven't taken any as I have been known to do many silly things when this liquid has entered my system. When I know I can sleep it off the following day, should there be any weird happenings again, I will have a go and hope the result will not have me resembling someone who has had a heavy night on the Guinness!

My chemo has been slightly increased again as my last cycle of a very reduced dose worked well without any stomach pain.

Mentally, I will feel happier in myself, thinking this higher dose will be attacking the cancer again.

When I was very ill in September I never thought I would go on to it again but, once things settle down, it feels as if the drug-taking isn't an option, it's a must.

We all know how the NHS appears to have money problems all the time, with cuts being constantly made in the hope of saving cash, but a new system in the day unit of putting name bracelets on daily chemo patients would seem an unlikely money-saving scheme.

Our names and date of birth are checked before treatment begins but as we are mostly well enough to answer correctly, these bracelets seem to be of little use.

I guess the person who thought this up had their reasons for doing so but I can't help thinking that, at the end of the financial year, the amount of plastic name tags used will mount up to a reasonable sum of money which could have been put to much better use.

As for the giggling I mentioned earlier, well that will continue up to December and probably beyond. You see, I have been invited to a Christmas reception hosted by - wait for it - the Queen! When the letter arrived I didn't for one minute believe it to be genuine so I accused many of my friends of joking at my expense! In the end I phoned the given number only to be answered with the words: "Buckingham Palace".

I was so taken back that I went into one of my muddled sessions and I ended up saying that I had this weird letter and was phoning up to see if it was true. Only I could manage to leave such an impression! I am allowed to bring one guest, who, of course, will be David. Ideally, I would like to ask for many more invites so that I could bring all of my friends, but I'm not so sure Liz (as she is known to her friends!) would oblige. A friend, however, will go to London with us for the day and will take K&F out for dinner after they watch us go in.

'Brave is not a word to describe how I am, but I am strong'

I just cannot believe this has happened, it is one of those extremely surreal moments in life that makes me think I've been back on the morphine for a while. Each time I look at the envelope which is post-marked "Buckingham Palace" I giggle and think: "Yes, it does have my name on it!"

I am so far unaware of how I came to be on the guest list; it says it is a reception to recognise people who have made a significant recent contribution to life. I would not class myself as being part of this group of people.

As to why I am will always be a mystery, but to say I feel so privileged doesn't start to portray how excited I am about it all. Now lead me to that new outfit and move over Posh and Becks!

Wear It Pink Day proved a huge success just over a week ago, with The Angel in Lavenham raising £150, helped by owners Roy and John rounding up the donations given to this amount. Corncraft equally had a fantastic day with their teas and coffee coming in with a great £115.

My friend Mandy's son, Sam, collected £55 from The Cock, in Lavenham, and Heeks, on Market Square in the village, who don't even know me, kindly joined in with the pink theme and raised £40.

What a generous day it was, with local people once again doing this breast cancer charity proud. Everyone I saw looked absolutely wonderful in pink.

And as for Allister in The Angel, well you were a vision in that salmon pink T-shirt!

I am sitting beside a beautiful vase of flowers which have been sent to me by Maria and family, and a very special angel doll and Irish cross from Mike (now a known voice to me on the phone).

With my present vocabulary, I am finding it very difficult to fully express my thanks to you all. I am not sure what I have done to receive such wonderful gifts. I am not actually anyone very special and am only capable of writing about my life as it now is.

Brave is not a word to describe how I am, but I am strong. However, I am no different from any other cancer sufferer.

Strength is something that automatically comes after a diagnosis, it doesn't matter what age, gender or cancer type, your mind will always be there when you need it most.

So, from my very basic understanding of life, come these simple but meaningful words: Thank you.

My charity cards seem to be going in the right direction - however the hospital I attend is unable to sell them due to various restrictions, which is a great shame. I will now spend this week trying to find other ways of selling them.

I have also been professionally advised against selling just packs of Christmas cards but to have Jill's different water-colours as a set. After Christmas, the cards can then remain being sold and will carry on making money for various cancer charities. The pack will be of eight cards with three Christmas ones included. The other five will be for everyday occasions. The cards will be printed to a very high quality and, in my opinion, will be just wonderful.

I was introduced to the wonderful word "man-flu" by my friend Mandy recently and now my husband is suffering from this condition.

Noises floating my way have given me an idea of my next project: contacting Mr Oxford to get this illness, already highly recognised by women everywhere, its own entry into all future dictionaries!

I love cosy nights at home and probably am one of the few people who loved the hour going back last weekend.

The difference in time has also brought me great joy as when I am in my car, I now know exactly what time it is.

I never worked out how to change my car clock back in March, which had me living all spring and summer at a different time to everyone else!

Rhona x

November 15, 2004: *Woodentops, wine and marathon man*

FROM the age of seven, I wanted to be an air stewardess, which I was lucky enough to do and love for a decade of my life.

However, when I used to sit at an even earlier age with my mum, watching *The Woodentops*, I never dreamt that, some 40 years later, I would become a member of that odd-walking family!

My bones are not behaving the way I would like them to. When I get out of bed or get up after sitting, they feel as if they are pieces of inflexible hardboard nailed together at the joints, just like the characters of this very old tiny tots' programme.

I wonder why I should remember this 1960s' lunchtime entertainment more than any other. Maybe I knew deep inside that one day I would become just like them!

I started my prescribed morphine but then, a few days later, I stopped it again. On my drug-taking days, although my cough eased slightly, as did the pain, all I did was sleep. When I was briefly awake, my mind didn't feel sharp, my eyes always felt tired

and my head felt as if it was on the spin cycle of a washing machine.

I don't want to spend my life like this so, after four days, sleeping beauty (mmm, yes me!) awoke not to find Sean Bean, but an untidy house instead.

As I have cancelled seeing many of my friends recently, I thought: "No, it is time to go back to lunching!"

I am not one to devour information about all the side-effects of medication since reading once that a particular drug could lead to suicidal thoughts!

But I suppose I should have known that morphine and wine DO NOT MIX, so it was my own fault when I became very ill after a small glass of the red stuff.

Although I don't drink very much at all now, I just fancied it at that particular time and didn't think twice about the lethal mixture. I paid the price for my indulgence with a spinning head and a huge hangover the following morning. I will never repeat that mistake but I still will never read about all the drug side-effects, as

I have enough problems without thinking myself into others. The less known, in this case, is better for the mind.

Last Thursday, an article in the EADT had friends ringing me telling me about Paul Excell, who was running the New York Marathon for me.

I could not believe it. What a huge honour. It is so very unbelievable that people are doing things like this for me.

Paul, I hope you raise lots of money, you deserve to. You must be a very special person to do something like this for cancer.

During one of my morning sleeps (actually every day now) I was woken at 11.40 with a phone call from Radio Suffolk. As many of you know, I spoke to Lesley Dolphin during October, which was Breast Cancer Awareness Month, so I had sent her an e-mail telling her about my soon-to-be-unveiled charity cards.

The call, therefore, wasn't a surprise, but the fact that I was asked to talk on air within 10 minutes was!

I had to admit straight away that I had been asleep just moments earlier and, with my morning brain, I wouldn't be too quick with any answers.

I asked if anyone could help sell the cards for me, so it was lovely when I received a phone call immediately afterwards from a lady in Ipswich who, ironically enough, has terminal cancer herself.

Maud's Attic, a well-known shop to many in Ipswich, has also very kindly offered its support with the cards.

If anyone else feels they could also help, maybe you could call me on 01787 375310 or e-mail me at rhonasdiary@btinternet.com

The above two contacts will also be used for those who would like to buy the cards when they are available.

Thank you.

Thankfully, David is fully fit again - just as well really as, when I kicked him at night to stop him snoring, he took no notice and all that happened was I ended up hurting myself instead!

Throughout the past five years, I have sworn by Echinacea. I have suffered fewer problems with my immune system, such as colds and other bugs, than I should with chemo.

During 1999, when I was on an extremely powerful chemotherapy drug (AC) I was healthier than I had been before the diagnosis, which I put down purely to this one-a-day herbal tablet.

'I never thought I would be around one year later to watch him'

When you are reading this today, I will have proudly watched my son march on Remembrance Sunday with the ATC.

I never thought when I wrote about this last year that I would still be around to watch him one year later. To me, this is the most important Sunday of the year and, as a child, I was always there on that cold, normally frosty morning (hasn't the weather changed?), in my Brownie or Guide uniform with my parents close by.

I find it all very emotional and this year was no different. On Thursday, November 11, at 11am, when Big Ben sounded on my radio and the two minutes' silence was observed, I sat by the side of my bed with thoughts running through my mind like everyone else who respected this memory.

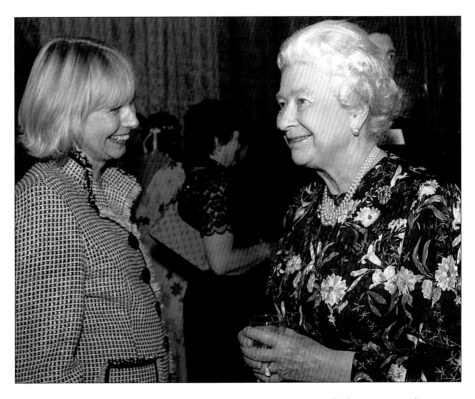

PROUD MOMENT: Rhona shares a joke with the Queen during a Christmas reception at Buckingham Palace. Rhona was one of 500 unsung heroes of charity and community work who were invited by the Queen to attend the reception in December 2004

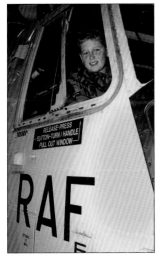

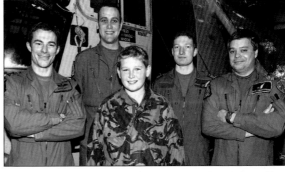

HIGH-FLYERS: Kristopher meets, from left, Flt Lt Dave Kay, Flt Lt John Tipper, Flt Sgt Will Harrison and Flt Sgt Steve Labouchardiere on a special visit to which he was treated by 22 Squadron, Wattisham Airfield. Left, Kristopher at the controls of one of the squadron's Sea King Search and Rescue helicopter. Kristopher's dream is to join the RAF

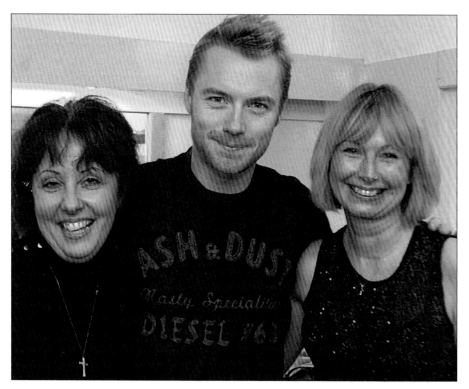

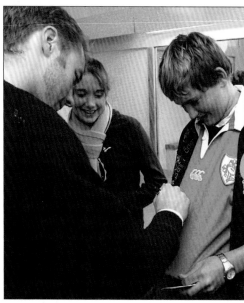

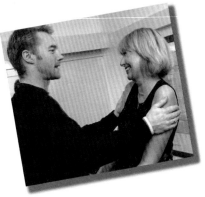

STARSTRUCK: Top, Rhona and Laini can't believe their luck - they're in the arms of Ronan Keating behind the scenes at his concert at Wembley Arena. Left, Ronan signs Kristopher's Ireland shirt and, above, Ronan and Rhona share a special moment

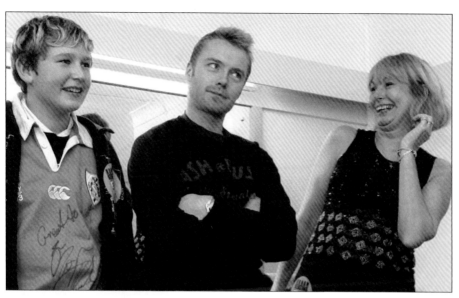

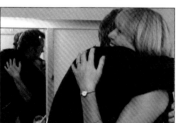

PRECIOUS MOMENTS: Top, **Rhona giggles as she and Kristopher chat with Ronan.** Left, **something to reflect on as Rhona gets a hug, and,** below, **it's just the ticket as Rhona shows off Ronan's message to 'The Jeffersons' backstage before the concert.** Below left, **Ronan rocks into action**

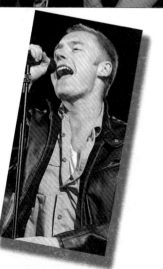

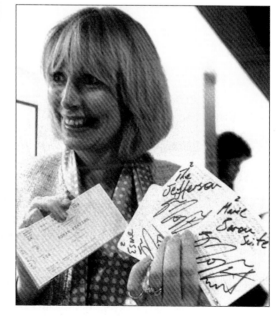

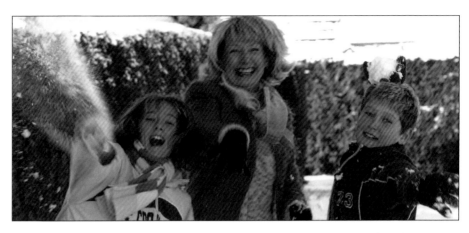

LOVE SNOWBALLS: Rhona enjoys some winter fun with Francesca and Kristopher

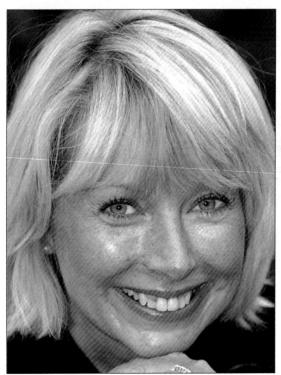

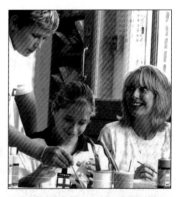

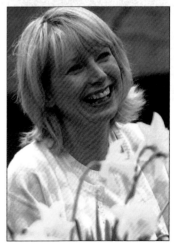

GREAT PERSONALITY: Rhona's wonderful winning smile radiates her warmth. Right, Rhona paints figures with Kristopher and Francesca during a visit to All Fired Up, Ipswich, and enjoys a spring day in her garden

I did think selfishly too, however where will I be here in a year's time? Who knows?

As I have been writing this there has been a silly programme on television, but something said made me look at it and laugh.

Apparently, according to this particular actor, nosebleeds qualify you for disabled parking nowadays!

So I hope I will stop having all the stares and glares when I park in these spaces, as I am well-known for my constant heavy nosebleeds. I'm not going to get into that great old debate again as I am one those who really gets upset when I see teenagers and people who are very able park in what is there to help those who are not.

Enough said (again!)

Rhona x

November 22, 2004: *Laughs between tears and tiredness*

I'VE had a very mixed week. The beginning, healthwise, was good, but at the end and as I write this, I've been back in bed again.

Wednesday was the day it all started to go wrong. A friend left at 7pm and just one hour later I was creeping slowly upstairs with various parts of my body niggled by sickly pain, which went on to give me another sleepless night.

Thursday was a bed day and by 8pm, having slept all day, I finally managed to get up, have some dinner and make a start on writing this. I am too greedy to ask for one wish - I would like two instead: to stay around for as long as possible with my family and to wake up one day, not tired and be allowed to do whatever I like without having to pay highly for it over the following 24 hours.

Reality hit me on Remembrance Sunday as I watched my son march with RAF Wattisham ATC. All parents are proud to see their offspring respect this war memory, so I wasn't any different to anyone else. But I spotted a family with their grown-up son, who had joined them for the church service dressed in his RAF uniform.

I wanted more than anything to be that family. I want to see my big son wear that uniform. I want to be that very proud mum standing beside her son, knowing he has achieved the career of his dreams and I want to see my son become a man. But because of a series of mishaps during recent years all of that will be taken away from me.

Why is life so unfair?

My main focus that chilly afternoon was that particular family. Throughout my life I have never felt more envious of anyone. Normality returned quickly as we left church, when Kristopher asked David to go into a pub and get him some pork scratchings and with that, a very sombre day for many reasons and for many people ended.

Having written about Paul Excell last week, it was great to finally get to talk to him last Monday about his run in the New York Marathon. He kindly sent me a photo of himself and his children, James and Jess. Up to now he has raised the fantastic amount of £2,100 and is hoping to reach the £3,000 mark for Breast Cancer Care (pretty impressive stuff, eh?).

Paul finished the race in a personal best time but without any toenails remaining. Having recently cracked one of mine in two, I can only start to imagine the discomfort he must be feeling (big ouch!)

"Special" is the word to describe you, Paul, and your family for taking time to show an interest in this horrible disease. Thank you for doing so. I hope that Paul's wife, Tracey, managed to get time to "do the shops" when they were there - there's nothing like a bit of culture in a woman's life!

Last Saturday, my friend Sue, her daughter Melanie, Francesca and myself went to see *Finding Neverland*. What a heartbreaker! The day started with me not being able to see where I was going, as we went into the screening five minutes into the trailers. I was completely blind and relying on my daughter to guide me to my seat. I really felt vulnerable being like this, due to the tumours in my eye.

It was only after my darling daughter shouted at me: "For goodness' sake, mum, you're wearing your sunglasses" that I realised it wasn't the cancer at all!

It was a film very close to home, which wasn't helped by the fact that fairies had quite a part in it.

Francesca, I could see, was also having little crying moments, but I think, as upsetting as it was, she will remember it for many years.

It is a very girlie, weepy film which left Sue and me without any make-up on our faces - it had all transferred to our tissues - and proved that our mascara wasn't that waterproof after all!

It is hard to say how much of a state we looked when we came out but the manager asked us if we were all right and could he do anything for us. When Sue told him we had just been to Neverland he looked slightly disturbed and left, saying he was concerned for our welfare.

Melanie and Francesca by this stage had "Oh no!" looks of horror on their faces but Sue and I just giggled our way into the ladies, knowing the mirror would show the true state of our tear-streaked faces. Believe you me, it wasn't a pretty sight!

It is a film any woman would love as it has it all; sentimentality, love, fairies, heartbreak - and Johnny Depp!

From next week my charity cards will be available to buy. I have had some great offers from people to help sell the cards and if anyone else thinks that they could get involved, could you please contact me on the following: rhonasdiary@btinternet.com or leave a message on 01787 375310 and I will call you back.

Apart from the printing costs all proceeds will go to various cancer charities, which will, I hope, amount to quite a good sum of money.

It's back to hospital again this week for my bone-drip. It is so unbelievable how this three-weekly drip comes around so quickly. My cough isn't any better, but then nothing else is either! I coped well again on this cycle of increased chemo, so I expect it will be a higher dosage again after this appointment.

The only thing I have against the oral drug is that I can often forget to take it, which is not a good idea. But then, during the past week I have also forgotten to eat, and on a visit to Tesco's for two items I couldn't remember why I was there and had to phone David to ask.

I know that carrot cake wasn't one of the two items, but it came home with me anyway!

Rhona x

November 29, 2004: *My new mates: Liz, Phil and Ronan*

NOW, what do you get when you mix together a fairy card, a Rhona's Diary cutting, a letter from Julian Ford (EADT features editor) and an input from Breakthrough Breast Cancer?

Only a foreword for my book written by the beautiful man himself - Ronan Keating! Now, did you really think when I was given

94

a "no" the first time of asking that I would let it go? Well of course not, so now I have a handwritten and well-thought-out piece of work, which I think will have to be framed and placed somewhere in my house so that everyone can see he is a good old mate of mine!

Along with Ronan's masterpiece came my official invite to meet Liz and Phil at the palace. Of course, all my friends are taking the mick out of me now. It still seems so unreal!

My hospital appointment, on Tuesday, came and went just like all the others, but there was one lovely difference this time - I was seen by a female doctor.

Naturally, over the years I have become accustomed to having male doctors examine my bits, but I wouldn't say I like it very much and each time I will lie with my eyes closed, trying to think of something else. However, on this occasion, I felt relaxed enough to speak during the examination. Even after six years, I'm afraid I am still very modest, even with the help of silicone. I can never see myself as an exhibitionist. Actually, as I am approaching my 44th birthday, I can hear you all shouting: "It's just as well!"

My blood count has lowered, which is why I think I am now so tired all the time. Apparently I could be in line for a blood transfusion soon. Good, as this could be what I need.

In the past two weeks I have left the house twice (not good, for those who lunch) and seem to spend my days sleeping.

On the phone I am very good at putting it on as if all is well, but in fact I am now a washed-out wreck! I am not eating, and there is nothing at all that I fancy, so I am living on toast with either jam or the healthier option of banana and that is it. My medication, therefore, has me feeling quite nauseous, as it is all falling on a sort of empty stomach.

As for my cough, well I would have been shot long ago if I had four legs!

All in all, I am not amused with myself right now. I expect it will get better, there will come a time when I will start to push myself harder again, but at the moment I prefer to sleep my days away. At least I get to forget it all that way.

"Tis the season to be spending, lunching and partying", so watch out friends, I will be back!

I am having a CT scan soon, but had to tell the doctor I wouldn't be available on December 7.

I was thinking, 'Oh please don't ask me why'. Could you imagine all the whisperings, if I had said: "I'm off to meet the Queen." There probably would have been a chorus of: "God love her, that brain tumour of hers has taken over her mind!"

My (charity) cards have arrived and I love them. After my recent requests for help, I now have many new-found friends willing to help sell them.

I did an interview on BBC Radio Essex during the past week, which had my phone ringing continuously. It is great knowing this step into the unknown of card production was the right thing to do.

As I previously mentioned, I was advised not to print only Christmas cards as they have such a short selling period, so we have come up with an "occasion pack", which will cover Christmas, Easter and all the

'In fact, I am now a washed-out wreck!"

95

other times when you need a card. All are blank in the middle, for your own wording, but the best of it is they work out at just 69p per card. A pack of eight will cost £5.50, of which, after printing and design costs, £4.20 will go to various cancer charities.

At present (until I can get my act together) the cards can be bought from the following places (a huge thank you to them for helping me): The Angel Hotel & Restaurant in Lavenham; Corncraft and The Summer House in Monks Eleigh; Maud's Attic, St Peters Street, Ipswich, EADT in Lower Brook Street, Ipswich.

Next week, I will have further addresses The cards can also be posted to anyone, by sending a cheque made out to "Rhona Damant", at 8 Whitehall Close, Gt Waldingfield, Sudbury, Suffolk, CO10 0XU.

Well, I'm off back to sleep; I might even dream that the blue-eyed Irish boy is singing just to me... aahhh!

Rhona x

December 6, 2004: *A fairy friend steps in*

REGRETTABLY, Rhona was unable to write her column this week as she has been admitted into hospital. So I will endeavour to write a brief, if not as humorous or as articulate, diary note on her behalf.

Unfortunately, the cancer in her lungs has spread and is causing her breathing difficulties. Having been admitted to hospital she has been put on oxygen and is now in a more comfortable position.

However, the hospital has now discovered a blood clot on her lung, so our determined "Irish Lass" is now also undergoing treatment for that.

Rhona is desperately fighting to get well enough to visit Her Majesty next week, and the hospital is doing what it can to get her strong enough to go.

They intend to give her portable oxygen and I am sure you will join with me in praying that she is well enough to attend.

With regards to the "Rhona Cards" I would like to assure you that all orders should still be addressed to Rhona at 8 Whitehall Close, Gt Waldingfield, Sudbury, Suffolk, and they will be despatched accordingly.

In closing, I would like to give praise to the most remarkable, determined and courageous woman I have ever met, someone who has been a true and loyal friend.

When Rhona organises all her friends for a little soiree it's a time of laughter and happy memories and sometimes we ask how can that be so.

You spend time with someone that you know is on borrowed time, and who you will lose sooner rather than later, and still have great laughter!

It's because Rhona makes it that way. Life on her terms - long may it be so.

'She is the most remarkable woman I have ever met'

A Fairy Friend x

96

December 13, 2004: *It s good to be home, I think!*

Hi, its me...the fat body inside a Dame's padded skin that doesn't seem to be quite me. Sorry but there won't be a huge amount from me this week, I am planning, however, to reveal ALL my secrets from my night at the palace next week.

I would love to be able to write all about the past week, but in all honesty, I am not very well and I am finding life extremely difficult right now.

With oral morphine and portable oxygen, along with a few other drugs here and there, I am now living life in a haze with what seems like cotton wool across my eyes at all times. My limbs feel alien and don't seem to be part of me any more.

It is oh so strange. There's a good song title. The feeling of isolation and the sense of feeling very frightened is quite overwhelming.

It has been good that since coming home from hospital I have not had a single moment alone. My friends are now rallying around at all times to make sure I have constant company. When I was given the news late on Monday that I would be allowed to go home, the usual state of euphoria didn't set in. Instead I was still sitting on my bed four hours later, not exactly wanting to leave. In seven days it's become my little safe area, knowing that no matter what happened I had one of my "Jefferson angels" close by my side.

The thought of returning to Waldingfield without my buzzer beside me sent me into formerly unknown shivers of apprehension throughout my body.

I expect I will become happier knowing that I can start to live on my own again without the need of someone being near. After all, only a week ago I was still this independent woman...I expect it is all a temporary measure of living out the quivering wreck of my life. The good - or maybe bad - news is that I have to go each week to Essex Rivers to have my blood checked, so I know that as soon as there is a further problem I shall be at the right place.

On Friday I went for a CT scan and a blood test. Merrily driving home with my friend Mandy, after shopping, I phoned up for the result expecting nothing to have changed in three days only to find the old red stuff was playing up again. So I'm on a different dosage to steady the blood flow from further clots and back on Tuesday for another test.

I've always wanted a second little holiday home (well, you know me and my dreams) well, I've got one now.

It's just 20 minutes down the road, daily changed white crisp bed linen on an electrical bed...what more could I want?

'My friends are now rallying round at all times'

I will have just celebrated another birthday (I'm sure I have had a second helping of that this year) so I deserve all that middle-age spread around my middle now. But it will have been a good day as the celebration will have been with all of those whom I love and have spent times with me when I needed them most.

On a final note...my cards. What can I say but "thank you" to everyone for sending them, they have been an unbelievable hit.

Many people have phoned me and left messages over the past week offering to help.

I hope most of you will have received your cards that have been ordered up to now, the latest requests from last week should be with you at the start of this week.

Please continue to send any orders to myself, which my friend Laini and I are sending out, to: 8,Whitehall Close, Gt Waldingfield, Sudbury, CO10 0XU. Telephone 01787 371823 or 01787 375310.

Other outlets now have been arranged by my fairy artist, Jill, so cards can also be purchased from:

Just a Thought in Head Street, Colchester; Something Special cafe and gallery, North Hill, Colchester; Adult education centre (Chris Wakeling) Colchester; The Bay Tree Restaurant, Connaught Avenue, Frinton; The Hospice Day Centre, Jackson Road, Clacton; Freeland Road post office, Clacton; Ardleigh Sports and Leisure Centre, Debham Road, Ardleigh.

Rhona x

December 20, 2004: *Life is a rollercoaster, you ve just got to ride it*

Rhona, can I ask you something? Are you frightened? Beacause I am. This is the question my friend Elizabeth asked me during the week. We have known each other 35 years plus so, for her, this was something she desperately needed to know.

I could hear her starting to get emotional and, a couple of times, I thought I was going the same way. But, for her, I managed to hold it together until after the phone call.

As for the answer, well no, I am not frightened. Nature, I now know, has a way of getting everyone ready for what we all know is in store at sometime in our future and I am lucky in that I have had a lot of time preparing myself and my family for it.

I am starting to feel very weary and feel the time is coming closer when I can allow my body to start to let go. I have taken my children from eight and nine to almost 14 and 15, and quite soon they will take on their own independent way of life.

I have achieved absolutely everything I could have wanted for my family, and more. Of course, I could be greedy and keep wanting (hot tub for instance!) but the memories held by everyone will be of good, funny and happy times, thankfully not sad.

Right, enough of that dying stuff. It's me, the person who went to the palace and couldn't quite work out the toilet!

Under my haze of morphine I am finding it more and more difficult to see. My vision is an absolute mess, talk about looking like a complete junkie! I'm sure people are now convinced I spend my free time in the less "salubrious" surroundings of Suffolk.

Lost track again, back to the "throne". All I can say is that it is very different! I am a hoverer when it comes to public toilets but couldn't quite manage this as it was the full width of the cubicle (not small) and looked like an old-fashioned wash basin which lifted up. The flush, well that was hidden and when I did finally find it under another walnut covering it didn't quite work!

Under medication it was all very difficult to work out and, in all, it took about 15 minutes to finally spend a penny. Needless to say I didn't go again!

I did do something very naughty though. Yep, you have guessed it. I took some toilet paper home for my friends (tacky or what?).

I was told by the Press office that I would be in the line-up to meet the Queen, which to my amazement I was quite calm about.

When I asked what I was meant to do and say, I was told that in 30 seconds a little lady in a lavender dress would be front of me, at which I looked in front of me, saw her and with some stupid voice came out with: "Hello".

When asked: "And who are you?", the same stupid voice said: "I'm Rhona Damant". But I managed to stop myself asking her who she was. I tell you, these drugs are something else.

We spoke about cancer and fundraising but it was only when I saw the footage on Anglia Television the following day that I realised she hadn't seemed to have been able to have got a word in edgeways. Even when she was talking to David I was still rabbiting on. At one stage I almost followed her as if to say: "Come back, I haven't finished yet!"

The fact that I even had an invitation sent to me was the highest honour I could ever wish for, but to have actually been presented to the Queen was unbelievable, so I could not believe how some people appeared to be there for their own glory. At times, little streaks of jealously even came through, which I would never have imagined could actually happen.

I had a lady (?) behind me kick me around my ankles (I still have the bruising to prove it), push me and throw her arm over my shoulder shouting something like: "Oh Queen, I want to shake your hand because you are a lovely woman!"

Someone else came over to ask me why I met her and then said: "Well, I have cancer. Why should you be allowed to meet her", followed up by a most distasteful face! Someone else didn't care too much that I was having a great conversation with Sophie Wessex and put his rather giant hand across my face to ask her if she had heard of the word "agriculture" because that is what he did. Honestly the embarrassment of my fellow breed (he was Irish). The thing is, he sounded just like my dad!

As I mentioned last week the highlight of the evening was my meaningful conversation with Sophie. She is beautiful in every way and, unknown to me and most others, she spends much of her time working for Haven, which is very similar to Breakthrough Breast Cancer. It was so nice to be able to communicate with someone who has dealt with this type of cancer and is also aware of the genetic side.

At the end of the evening we had stomachs very full of very rich canape food. At 8.30pm we left to get into our car, which was parked at the palace, and at 8.50pm we were sitting at MacDonald's with a hot chocolate and a hot apple pie. I know how to live! But there you go, that's reality for you!

'With a whoosh of magic dust, I was the old me again'

Since the palace, I have been a fairy at my Christmas open house which ended up being an almost 12-hour party.

I had been very down after my week in hospital immediately before, so my party could have gone either way. But at 11.30am, on December 12, I put on my fairy dress, followed by my wings and a tiara and with a whoosh of magic dust, I was the old me again. And I've stayed that way for most of the week. I had this idea that I would buy fairy wands for every man, which I did, and throughout that day each male at my party either held their wand, had it in their shirts or trousers - and when it was time to leave they still had them.

Throughout the day we had 97 friends so

that came to much wand-holding. So thank you to all my male friends for allowing me to be really very stupid that day!

It has been a week of constant hospital trips and it looks like it will continue for a little while as my blood is being just plain nasty. It will not regulate itself, so the clotting side is turning into a nightmare. One day it is too thin, the next too thick.

I am now getting quite used to constant blood tests but also I am getting to spend quite a lot of time in my safe comfort zone of the hospital.

As it stands this week, I have two definite appointments with, most likely, another one on Christmas Eve and then maybe a four-day break but back to see my friends on the Wednesday again.

For the first time in as long as I can remember we have not planned anything over Christmas and I am looking forward to it all very much. I can get up when I want, eat, drink, sleep whenever I want and it will all be with just my little family.

I have had a cross-match blood test taken just in case I need a top-up before Christmas. I hope whoever has donated it has had the silliest season this year, as I could do with having a 95% alcohol content rate, leaving me just 5% to sort out myself!

I'm off now for a lie down in a darkened room as I'm going to meet Ronan Keating on Wednesday night. The things people have to do in life!

So on that note, merry Christmas everyone. Enjoy your day as much as possible and don't hold back. Do whatever you want to do. After all, it's too late to be good for Santa!

Rhona x

December 27, 2004: *Still in shock from the last few months*

'TWAS the night before Ronan, and all through the house not a creature was stirring, except for Rhona Damant! I couldn't sleep and the last time I had butterflies in my stomach like that was on the eve of my O-levels.

My "Fairy friend" (who wrote my column for me when I was in hospital), Laini, came with me, Kristopher and Francesca.

I am not sure who was more giggly when the time came for one of the top moments of my life. The most amazing thing happened though - I was lost for words (a first in 44 years!). I just couldn't stop looking at this gorgeous man. He told me I looked amazing which, as you can imagine, just made my night, week, month!

We spoke about the foreword he has written for my book. He asked me to send him a copy and I had to sign it. Isn't it funny? Just before I met him he was a celebrity who I only watched on television and now look: he is my new best friend - I expect he will be inviting me to Dublin next (dream, dream!)

He signed coasters for the children and also for my "Jefferson angels" from the hospital and the chemo nurses, but then he said: "I can do better than that" and signed some programmes for us.

On mine he wrote: "2 Rhona, your strength amazes me, God bless you, Ronan Keating x."

I am in fairyland and I think I will remain there for a long time. Our meeting was not rushed, and he genuinely seemed very happy to be there with us. As he left, I got my much-wanted kiss and a huge hug.

No amount of morphine could ever put me this high.

It got even better during the concert, when he sang the line "I love you" from one of his songs and looked straight at me. I know that was meant just for me . . . as if he would say it to anyone else!

100

I am still in shock about everything that has happened in the last few months. I am just a good old Irish girl who was brought up on huge amounts of potatoes and learnt to drive with more cows on the road than cars.

I started writing this column for women like me who needed plain English answers to their questions, not all the medical jargon which comes with a cancer diagnosis. If I had been told back then that the diary would have a huge following, a book would be written, I would have my own charity cards, make large amounts of money for charity, be presented to the Queen and meet Ronan, I would never have believed it!

But all of this has happened for some reason. It has also given me a purpose in life, apart from being a mum and a wife.

It excites me when I get letters from people who have gained some sort of strength from what I write and the money raised all goes forward in the hope that one day a cure may be found, obviously not in my generation but, please God, for the next one.

2005 will most certainly bring my death, but it is also going to be an exciting year and when I am not around I hope my friends and children will carry on raising money. My cards will continue, with a change of designs replacing the Christmas ones.

I am still having dreadful problems with my blood, or my INR to be precise. INR stands for International Normalised Ratio, which is a measure of how much longer it takes blood to clot when an anticoagulation is used. So if the reading is 2.0, the blood is taking twice as long as normal to clot. The ideal reading is around 3.5 but mine is only 1.6 (not good).

I am now on 3mg a day of warfarin. My consultant would like me to go back on injections but I am not too keen on this idea, so presently I am allowed to continue with the tablets. But I think if my blood does not

change very soon, the dreaded needle will be introduced again (help!). I am having my blood checked every three days but hope to have a four-day break over Christmas. Should there be a problem, I will be able to go back to my second home.

Warfarin is an amazing drug as it stops blood from clotting within the blood vessels. It is also used to stop existing clots from getting any bigger and stops parts of clots breaking off and forming emboli (material which lodges in the pulmonary circulation, impeding the blood flow). Anticoagulations can prevent the clotting of blood and prevents formation of harmful clots in blood vessels by decreasing the blood's ability to clump together. During the week I had two instances with my cough that demonstrated how some people can be nice and others quite hurtful. One day, when I was out and coughing quite badly, a women said: "Can't you do something about that cough? It really is irritating."

'The money raised goes forward in the hope that a cure will be found'

I don't know what stopped me from telling her why I was coughing but it was quite obvious to her that I wasn't well. All she was worried about, though, was my cough annoying her!

A few days later, I was in a beautiful shop, called The Bay Tree, in Colchester, and again I was coughing badly. On this occasion, a lovely man went and found some mints to try to ease the fluster which I was starting to get in. When you read this, Christmas will be over. I hope you all had a great time. We will have had our family time, which could have been spoilt for us, as Kristopher's main present was stolen. I ordered an ipod at the beginning of November, but when I phoned two days before Christmas to see why it hadn't arrived I was told it had been delivered on December 2. Now, as I was in hospital, there wouldn't have been anyone here to sign for it.

Our New Year, like Christmas, will be very quiet. That is how I want it. With how my health is going, it will be my last one and I don't, therefore, want to share my family with anyone else. Then, after that, it will be busy, busy with my fundraising again.

This has been an unbelievable year for me and it has been down to all of you, with all of your good wishes and prayers, not forgetting all those hard-earned pennies.

I wish everyone of you the most wonderful 2005.

May it be happy, but above all healthy.

Rhona x

P.S: My charity cards are available at £5.50 a pack from 8 Whitehall Close, Great Waldingfield, Sudbury CO10 0XU. Make cheques payable to Rhona Damant.

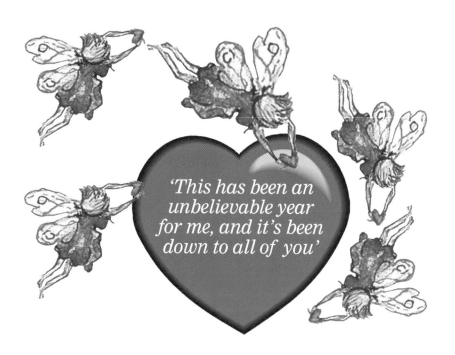

'This has been an unbelievable year for me, and it's been down to all of you'

Rhona's helpful hints

Travel insurance: Try Freedom Insurance Services Ltd. No 13-year-old boys working here - ring 0870 7743760.

CancerBACUP: For lots of information - www.cancerbacup.org.uk

Nuisance phone calls: If you do not want phone calls from someone trying to sell you insurance, which can be upsetting, ring 0845 0700707 to register your name to stop them.

Holidays: Before flying, phone the airline and ask for a preboard. It may cost you a doctor's letter but it takes away all the strain and stress of queuing to board your flight. If the flight is a long one ask for a wheelchair as this does away with all the standing when you are waiting to go through immigration.

Sunbathing: If radiotherapy has recently taken place you must use a high-factor sun lotion as your skin will burn from the previous effects of treatment.

Flight socks: A must for cancer patients when flying - very glamorous!

The Body Shop: They are understanding and good to go to when the eyebrows leave - they will teach you how to 'feather' new eyebrows in with the right colour for your face.

Anaesthetic cream: Ametop is wonderful stuff - it's numbing so you can't feel the needle go in.

Radiotherapy: For the side-effects, E45 cream is just the best!

Chemotherapy: For the sickness, fresh ginger juice from the health shop mixed with spring water. Also try flat lemonade.

Hair: Before you find it on your pillow, have it shaved - it eases much of the distress. Buy lots of fabric and, if like me you can't sew, get a friend to do it! All you need is a triangle and it can be tied in many ways. If, like me, hats are the chosen accessory and someone stares throughout having a meal out, go up to them at the end, thank them for spoiling your night and then lift your hat up. Tell them that's why you are wearing a hat - and they'll never do it again!

To become a Marsden patient: If you want a second opinion from the top cancer hospital ask your doctor to refer you. Not all Marsden patients are private and you will get the same treatment on the NHS!

If you have children: Hospices often have counsellors who can come to your home and befriend your child. Their feelings can come out by using puppets pretending that it is the toy that is sad, not the child. Books can also be used to write down feelings, with drawings to help, or buy a dog like we did when the kids were older.

Echinacea: A must for immune systems and as a general pick-me-up against germs when you are low.

Benefits: Don't feel too proud to ask for what you are entitled to. I was, but then someone reminded me how I have worked all my life...enough said! My MacMillan nurse sorted this out for me.

Disabled parking: Again, my MacMillan nurse sorted this out for me and it is a vital part of my life if I have to go out during oxygen days and when my bones are not in working order.

Build-up: Lemon and lime flavour. Put in the blender, add some ice cream and mix up to a brilliant milk shake when the appetite level isn't too high.

Bach Rescue Remedy: For those uncertain moments when the nerves tend to take over. Four drops of this on your tongue - it's amazing!

Hospital transport: I used to get a hospital car that took David and I to the Marsden. It was arranged through my GP and saved me so much energy and David so much stress!

And finally...

It is Friday January 21, 2005, 9.40pm and the forecast is for winter weather over the next few days. Great, as I love snow, but equally great as I am now just starting to put pen to paper for the summing up last chapter of my "dream" - *Sit Down and Stop Laughing.*

To be able to write this with what I hope will be Christmas card scenes around me will be the final piece of magic needed to finish off my very magical year.

I have decided to handwrite this, my final ending, as it will be personal to me and to those who will want to remember my scrawl in years to come. My old mate Ronan has kindly handwritten his foreword so I thought, what better way to finish it? I know it can't all be printed in my writing, but what is allowed will be just fine by me.

To have a life with cancer is no mean dream, but to have had the life I have had since December 11, 1960 until, I hope, much further into the year of 2005 has been one that most people would be happy with. I had a lovely childhood, achieved my dream career, followed my dreams (which everyone should do) married a wonderful man, who loved me for what I was (a nightmare!) and ended up with two beautiful children.

Many people have thought my book would be about my life, but hey, how boring would that be? It would definitely be worse, I'm sure, than looking at friends' holiday photos. You know when that yawn is about to happen but somehow you manage to turn it into a smile instead.

As all books need excitement, I've spiced mine up with talking very openly about living with the "Big C". This has been the theme of *Rhona's Diary*, as printed each Monday in the *East Anglian Daily Times.*

As I write this, I have just come out of hospital again, having just been in there six weeks earlier and eight weeks before that. This means one thing. Unfortunately, my cancer is starting to hit hard and furiously so now the time has come to tie up all those lose ends in my life, sit back and enjoy the days ahead as much as possible .

I haven't as yet bought all the cards I want for the children (a birthday card for each year up to 21, exams, good luck cards, driving tests, engagement and wedding cards).

Their memory books haven't been finished either but this book is my dream and it will be there for them as a reminder of their lives. I hope, more than anything, it will make them proud of their mum and maybe, in time, they will say: "Yep, she was all right, our mum."

So, a quick story of my life then. Well, I am the only child of two very Irish parents who were your real-life Darby and Joan. I used to think it was so disgusting to be so much in love. Mind you, it was also quite sad as their cosy little life didn't allow for others to gain entry.

As any other Irish child did, I grew up with a main menu of stews, always more potatoes than meat. I never seemed to have many friends throughout my early life as that would have been an intrusion and that was a big no-no in our family of three.

Church was a main feature, which meant that each Sunday I would get to dress up in my best dress, straw hat, white lace gloves, white socks and shoes - and in my little plastic bag I would always have my white Bible.

I would think to the outside world we were the perfect little family but underneath, heartbreak had played a big part in family life. My cousin had died of leukaemia, which was followed by the death of her baby brother.

Twelve months after Patricia's death a

surprise baby named Rhona Stephanie Sylvia Hutchinson arrived in the world and apparently looked very similar to my cousin throughout her early years.

My mum loomed from the stereotypical, large but close-knit Irish family. And with families of that size, as per usual, there happened to be some who thought of themselves as rather regal-like, whereas others couldn't give a damn.

My granddad was a music teacher but liked the old whisky too much so could be a great embarrassment to the snotty ones (one aunt played violin for the London Philharmonic Orchestra).

Although the aunts and uncles had the same background they all went different ways in their lives - some better than others - but they did have a very happy family.

My only memory of my lovely old red-nosed granddad was when my aunt's posh friends came to stay. He would drink out of a tin mug (brown lemonade, as we had then in Ireland, tasted the best from this). He would tear a piece of sheeting apart, use it as a hankie and shout to my grandma: "Hey Jinnie, where is the eiderdown?" while shaking this disgusting old thing around.

He was a very clever man but wouldn't suffer fools gladly, and it is due to old Sam that I have the personality I have. I am a person who cannot stand someone who puts it on, if you know what I mean. I can't for the life of me understand why some need to add certain pretentious stories to their lives. Why can't everyone be normal and be done with it. What a strange old world we now seem to live in.

As with most adults, my summers are remembered to have been long, hot, sunny and perfect.

Early holidays were modest, but as I grew up, Ireland suddenly didn't seem to be too far away from the Continent, so we became the more out-going Irish traveller. My life,

looking back on it, did seem to be quite idyllic. However, I can still feel the sting of the wooden spoon on the back of my legs - oh,how it hurt. It was only my mum who was the user. My dad used to dry the tears - what are dads like with their little girlies?

In fact, I was known as his little lady baby, a name Francesca took over when she was born.

Thirteen was the age I was considered to be grown up so I was taken to Paris to find the culture. It was a wonderful spring holiday and one of which memories are made. Six months later my mum was dead and I was grown up for good.

Aged just 45, my beautiful, brilliant, remarkable mum had died from the unmentionable - breast cancer.

After returning from France, she started to experience major pain in her hips and just weeks later she was silently diagnosed in the Royal Victoria Hospital in Belfast. In many ways, my her breast cancer hasn't changed much from hers: most still die. Hard to think of that, isn't it?

Her surgery was just as mutilating as mine. Thankfully she never had to lose her self-confidence by losing her hair (just about the worst thing for a woman with cancer. I absolutely hated it.)

My mum went into what can only be described as an isolated institution called Montgomery House. She would go on a Monday morning and return on a Friday afternoon. However, her whole weekend was spent being sick and often crying out in pain.

Like me, she suffered from blood clots but lived on daily warfarin. If though, she had been told she needed daily injections of the lovely Clexane, it wouldn't have upset her like it does me. My mum was never a wimp, unlike her daft daughter.

In Ireland, funerals normally take place the following day (well, they did then anyway) so we never had the long waiting game to bury her. That dreadful day was a wet autumn day and was the biggest funeral I have ever known.

It was such a huge surprise when I walked in with my dad, as I couldn't understand where all the people had come from. With it being a sort of unexpected death (very few people knew she had cancer) and also because she was quite young, it was amazing how many people came out of the woodwork (actually, the Irish are quite a nosy breed!).

From that night until many months later, my dad had to sleep on my bedroom floor (I obviously wasn't really that grown up after all).

Two months after my mum's death my dad had a heart attack. He returned to my floor when he came home from hospital, but many things changed.

I discovered that my mum had asked my dad to finish her life early for her to escape her life of pain and she wanted him to go with her. My dad did neither as he knew he had to bring me up.

After his heart attack he started on what seemed to be a dislike for me, finishing up with days of completely ignoring me. This, in his mind, was my punishment for being around and so stopping him from being with his gorgeous wife.

So, from being quite immature, this time the quick growing up was here for good - another side of my personality strength.

I suddenly had to look after myself, a house, a dog, continue my studies and hope that everyday my dad, who had turned to drink and religion, would go back to loving me as he once did.

Thankfully, he did, in time, go back to his old ways of being my lovely dad and although I never stopped loving him, I think his love for my mum was more then than it was for me.

What was going on around me at that horrible time made me mature beyond my years. I did eventually become his little girl again, initially not as wonderful, but we got there.

I never felt the need to rebel in my teens as many of my friends did. However, I always seemed to fall in and out of love about every week. My first real love happened when I was 14 - oh, the hurt when the big romance ended. Our involvement then consisted of phone calls and letters. There was none of this going out with someone then - what an innocent life I led.

I studied hard for my O-levels and managed 10 excellent grades with an A in geography - only because I fancied the teacher rotten!

I met a footballer when I was 16 and we remained together for seven years and were engaged for two. I had chosen two careers in my life - one to study law and the second to be an air stewardess. In the end, I chose the second and that was the cause of our break-up.

Most little girls dream of having the glamour of this (or lack of it at times) and I was very lucky to have lived this dream. I travelled the world for almost 11 years and felt privileged to have loved my life as much as I did. In all honesty I think I deserved it a little too as a part of my life really hadn't been very pleasant at all. It's a job that I wouldn't like to do now (not that I could, I suppose - but Rhona, just think about it, who wants a fairy when they are 44?)

In 1984 I had the opportunity to live in the Middle East and live and fly tax-free for two years. After four months of living this selfish life I met David, the man who would go on to put up with so much in later years. Being in the Gulf (Bahrain, to be exact) took me to even more places around the world but I still can't understand what on earth drew me to every tacky ornament going which, in turn, I would give to my old dad. He, in turn, loved them. Isn't it terrible what we daughters often have to put our parents through?

1984-6 gave me the independence I needed to carry me through my life, so it was the best thing I ever did in more ways than one. I also had the chance to save money (I learned to spend David's from an early stage) which in 1987 helped D and myself set up home.

After much travelling, I became Mrs Damant on Saturday, April 2, 1988. We had a wonderful wedding at Hintlesham followed by a reception in the glorious setting of Seckford Hall, Woodbridge.

My dad, although sad at handing his daughter over to an Englishman, was at the same time happy in his heart as he knew I had married the right man. At one time in our relationship when we briefly had a break, good old dad made me get back in contact and talked me into marrying him!

Flying off on honeymoon was something I didn't care too much for, so David booked us on the Orient Express visiting Paris and Venice. Now that was glamour.

Unfortunately, I suffered too many miscarriages, so I gave up my flying career. My boy arrived early into our lives on April 26, 1990, very quickly followed by his little sweet-pea sister on May 15, 1991.

David decided by then our family was complete, even though I would have liked a third. But on that occasion he would not give in to me. So we remained the Damant family of four.

The first year of the family's life was hell and I hated it. I even almost went back to British Airways at one stage, the children were such hard work. I swear it was worse than having twins as both, although close in age, were always at different stages. Sleep

never happened for us and we turned into exhausted wrecks. Even my poor old dad had to come over to stay for a long period to help us feel more like human beings.

The following year my dad suffered health problems so we moved him over from Belfast to live with us. It changed our lives so much that I even went back to work part-time to give us a little extra for luxuries and little girls' pretty frilly dresses! After a year of living with us his health improved enough for him to move into his own flat five minutes away.

Our family life ran on like anyone else's - ups and downs, good and bad days. On November 27, 1998 my dad babysat for us. On November 28 he died unexpectedly. David found him and from that day my life changed. I could not accept his death and often at first could not get through the first five minutes of the day without tears. It wasn't until the following summer that my grief started to subside.

The middle of August brought my diagnosis of an 11cm tumour in my right breast and the rest, as they say folks, is history!

Cancer again changed another life and another close family forever. As you know, I did not start to write about my life with cancer until the terminal diagnosis came, but Round One brought with it all the gruesome side of cancer - severe chemo, mastectomy, reconstruction and five full weeks of radiotherapy, along with sickness like I had never known, the loss of my once-thick hair and a weight of only six stone.

In March 2003 I was in remission and all thoughts of cancer seemed to go behind me. June 2003, after many mistakes, brought the final chapter of my life...and the rest you have just been reading about.

Well, my writing for my book is almost at an end but the snow never happened - however, it has been so cold and I have managed to sit in front of the odd log fire or two. My column-writing, I hope, has given you an insight into how life doesn't stop even when cancer appears. There can be an awful lot of living when it does happen and dreams can be fulfilled.

The bad side is you just never know when that time-bomb will explode - the good side of losing your hair is that there won't be any bad hair days for several weeks!

To those of you out there like me and to those who aren't, remember that this life is worth living as full as possible because we won't get a second chance to try it.

I give all my thanks to the very special people at the *East Anglian Daily Times* who have made my dream of writing a book come true, especially Dominic Castle, John and Sheena Grant, Roger Hall, Richard Peace, Mike Oliver, Dave Perkins and Paul Copsey.

I also thank the many readers who have sent me cards and letters of encouragement and kept me going through the bad days.

Thank you for all the presents I have been sent, thank you for thinking I have been worth it.

Thank you to all my many friends who have helped me lunch and listened to the tears when the "happy pills" haven't worked, and to my lovely David, Kristopher, Francesca and Lily-Dog who have just been there!

Of course life will continue for everyone when I have left to grow some fairy wings and fly off to be with my mum and dad, but please try to never forget me.

Rhona x

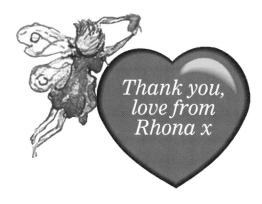

Thank you,
love from
Rhona x